THE HYPERBARIC CHAMBER: SCIENCE, NOT MIRACLE

Dr. Nina Subbotina

Alexandria Library
MIAMI

© 2011 Nina Subbotina
ALL RIGHTS RESERVED
No portion of this book may be reproduced, stored in a retrival system, or transmitted in any form except for brief quotations in critical review or articles, without the written permission of the author.

ISBN: 978-1494361051
Library of Congress Control Number: 2011903216

www.alexlib.com/notmiracle
samhas@hipercamaras.com.ar

www.alexlib.com

Content

- Oxygen and the Hyperbaric Chamber — 5
- Chronic Wounds or Non Healing Ulcers — 15
- Diabetic Foot Ulcer — 21
- Gas Gangrene and Others Infections — 32
- Severe trauma — 40
- República de Cromagnon's Tragedy: Smoke and Toxic Gases — 51
- Radiation Necrosis — 67
- Aseptic Bone Necrosis — 83
- Sudden Deafness and Acoustic Trauma — 88
- Neurological Disorders — 97
- Children with Autism — 106
- Cerebral Palsy — 113
- Contraindications, Side effects and Complications — 120
- Anti-Aging — 125

Oxygen and the Hyperbaric Chamber

Jules Verne (1828-1905) a French writer known as the author of novels such as *Twenty Thousand Leagues Under the Sea*, pioneer of the science-fiction genre, prophesying many inventions of the modern technology, also wrote a story about oxygen, this almost miraculous gas, which keeps us alive.

In *Doctor Ox's Experiment*, Verne describes the lethargic life of the inhabitants of hypothetical city of Quiquendone, situated in the heart of Flanders. This begins to change when Doctor Ox, a scientist, suggests to install a promising system of artificial lighting by means of "oxyhydrogen" gas. The town's authorities accepted the offer of better lighting at no charge. Dr. Ox's hidden interest is however not lighting, but large scale experiment on effect of oxygen on plants, animals and humans.

He uses electrolysis to separate water into hydrogen and oxygen. The oxygen is being pumped to the city causing accelerated growth of plants, and excitement in animals and humans. The people, who lived in somnolent state, begin to

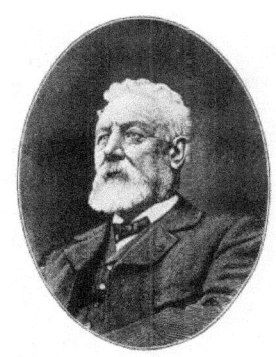

Jules Verne

> The modern hyperbaric chamber is an enclosure within which pure oxygen is breathed while the entire body is subjected to pressure greater than the normal atmospheric.

awake; they become more active and almost declare a war to their neighbors.

Jules Verne finishes the book with a rhetorical question: "Are virtue, courage, talent, wit, imagination, are all these remarkable qualities or faculties only a question of oxygen?"

What Is the Famous Oxygen?

Oxygen is the gas of the life. We cannot survive even five minutes without oxygen. It is a drug to which we all are "addicted". The blood transports oxygen from the lungs to the whole body in two forms: bound to hemoglobin (the main protein of red blood cells) and dissolved in plasma (liquid part of the blood).

Nowadays we know that oxygen is not only a substance to breathe and to produce energy, but it has other functions, in particular, it enables the white blood cells to kill the bacteria and other microbes that enter our organisms, so oxygen helps to protect us against infections.

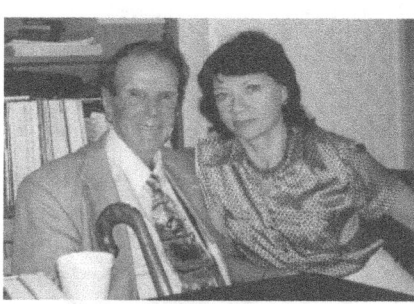

Doctor Neubauer and the author in the Ocean Hyperbaric Center, Lauderdale by the Sea, Fl.

Oxygen is used to treat critically ill patients. Sports records are achieved by athletes whose muscles are able to use more oxygen for energy production.

The Hyperbaric Chamber

The humanity acquired a very powerful therapeutic method discovering how to apply oxygen in hyperbaric form. Some people think that hyperbaric oxygen is miraculous. "It is not miracle, it is science", used to say Doctor Neubauer, who was a director of the Ocean Hyperbaric Center, in Fort Lauderdale, Florida, and who during decades dedicated his efforts to hyperbaric medicine.

The hyperbaric (hyper - greater, bar - pressure) chamber is a closed usually metallic device in which the body is held under a pressure greater than the atmospheric. Three and a half centuries have now passed from the invention of the hyperbaric chamber. In 1662 an English clergyman, Henshaw supposed

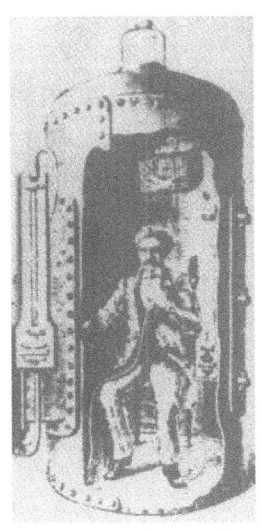

Paul Bert (father of hyperbaric physiology) in an experimental chamber.

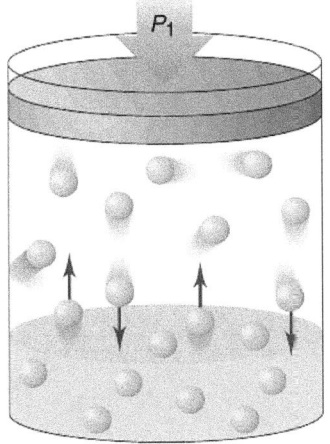
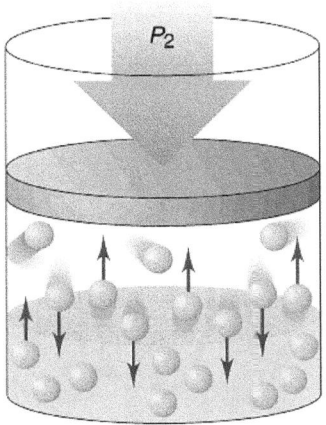

As higher the external pressure, the greater amount of gases dissolved in a liquid.

WHEN BREATHING AIR		
	If the body is subjected to:	Oxygen dissolved in 100 ml of blood
	Normal Atmospheric Pressure (1ATA)	0.3 ml
	In the Chamber to 2ATA	0.6 ml
	In the Chamber to 3ATA	0.9 ml

THE HYPERBARIC CHAMBER. SCIENCE, NOT MIRACLE

WHEN BREATHING PURE OXYGEN		
	If the body is subjected to::	Oxygen dissolved in 100 ml of blood
	Normal Atmospheric Pressure (1ATA)	2.1 ml
	In the Chamber to 2 ATA	4.5 ml
	In the Chamber to 3 ATA	6.8 ml

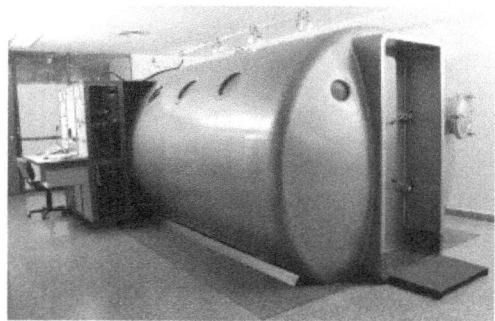
Outside of a multiplace chamber.

that under certain conditions, being put under a pressure greater than the normal atmospheric a sick person can feel better. First it was only air under pressure that was applied in the hyperbaric chambers. At the beginning of the 20th century, during the construction of the Panama Canal, the chamber was used for the first time in cases of caisson disease; we now call it decompression sickness, which occurs when the surrounding pressure falls abruptly. The idea of oxygen breathing to treat the decompression sickness in divers was studied from 1897 and tested and recommended in the 1930's.

During the 1950's the great Dutch physician-surgeon Doctor Boerema made an outstanding observation when he replaced all the blood of piglets that inhaled oxygen in a hyperbaric chamber by physiological solution. The skin of the animals became white instead of pink, but they were alive without blood, conserving all their energy, something impossible outside the hyperbaric chamber. Due to certain laws of physics, the greater pressure to which the body is subjected within the chamber permits a greater amount of inhaled oxygen to be dissolved in our blood and tissues. This increases the partial pressure of oxygen in the entire organism.

Since the publication of Doctor Boerema's article "Life without blood", hundreds of thriving medical studies have expanded the application of the hyperbaric oxygen

The Hyperbaric Chamber. Science, Not Miracle

to the treatment of different pathologies. The concept of "hyperbaric oxygen." abbreviated as HBO, HBO2 and "hyperbaric oxygen treatment" shortened also as HBOT have entered the medical vocabulary.

Monoplace and Multiplace Chambers

The modern hyperbaric chambers can incorporate a single person, they are commonly called "monoplace", or several people within a "multiplace". Chambers are generally cylindrical, resembling a little submarine. The monoplace chambers are pressurized directly with oxygen and the multiplace with air. Nowadays the best clinics in Europe and U.S. have available rectangular chambers, similar to common rooms which lessen the fear of confinement.

When the patient is placed in a monoplace chamber, the door is closed, oxygen begins to enter and the pressure rises. The patient breathes that same oxygen that is used to pressurize the chamber. A multiplace chamber is pressurized with atmospheric air, and the patients breathe oxygen delivered by masks.

The therapeutic effect in both types of chambers is the same.

Patient inside the Chamber

The design of the majority of monoplace chambers is such that the patient is laid down, whereas in the multiplace chambers patients can be seated or laid down, depending on

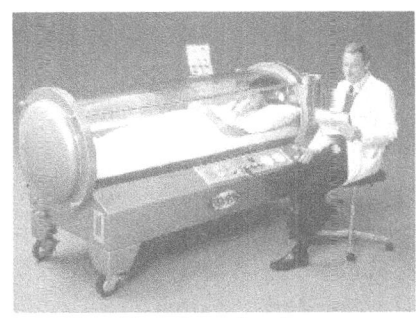

Monoplace chamber
Courtesy of Sechrist Industries, Inc.

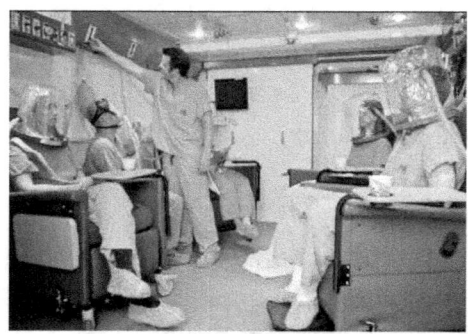

Interior of the Multiplace hyperbaric chamber Fink DL8. Courtesy of Lin Weaver, MD, Intermountain Medical Center, Murray, Utah

state of health. The hyperbaric personnel is always striving for the most comfortable position for patients, while providing the best professional care and conditions. Generally hyperbaric treatments take between 60 and 90 minutes.

The pressure increases gradually reaching the prescribed settings in about 10-15 minutes. As the pressure increases a patient can suffer a slight pain in the ears. This happens due to the pressure difference in the chamber and the middle ear. The effect is similar to what we feel traveling in an airplane, or when one changes altitudes during driving, climbing mountains or diving.

We teach patients to equalize those pressures by swallowing often enough to compensate the difference. Additionally this effect can be alleviated by trying to exhale air, keeping mouth and nose closed (Valsalva's maneuver). Another method is using a jaw movement similar to chewing gum, opening and closing mouth or yawning.

Before hyperbaric treatment a thorough examination of each patient is performed. As a routine, a thorax x-ray, and an electrocardiogram are requested. Some patients with previous problems in ear, nose and paranasal sinuses need an additional otolaryngologist' consultation. Others might require something else which will indicate the hyperbaric doctor un order to discard the presence of contraindications.

From the outer control post of the multiplace chamber the interior is checked by a video system. Also there are view ports or chamber windows that permit a direct visualization of the patients.

Safety of Hyperbaric Facility

Oxygen by itself is not flammable, but it is necessary for combustion to take place. Its excess facilitates the ignition, for this reason all hyperbaric medicine services have strict safety measures to avoid fires and explosions. Within the chamber the electrical and electronic devices, cell phones, matches, cigarettes, lighters, and other ignition sources are prohibited.

When the health care professionals need to enter or exit a pressurized multiplace chamber without pressure loss, the airlock, a small, hermetic, and contiguous to the chamber space is used. The airlock is separated from the main chamber by a door. The pressure in the airlock can be controlled independently from the pressure in the main chamber. If another assistant in the chamber is needed, he enters the airlock, the pressure rises until the level of the main chamber, the door is opened and the tender enters the main chamber.

The Hyperbaric Medicine as a Specialty

Patients who receive treatment in a hyperbaric chamber may be critically ill. Some arrive in comatose state, for example, poisoned with carbon monoxide, suffering gas gangrene or victims of a diving accident. The hyperbaric doctors must be qualified to provide care for a variety of conditions.

As of current, the university educational program has yet to include this specialty, although there are internationally recognized postgraduate courses of hyperbaric medicine. The professionals who evolve in this area must know the effects of pressure changes on the human organism, the physics of gases, biochemistry of oxygen and its reactive species commonly known as free radicals. Additionally physicians should be aware of the operation of the hyperbaric chambers, protocols of treatment for every type of pathology, management of possible medication changes in some patients and the multidisciplinary strategy to apply in every case.

Chronic Wounds or Non Healing Ulcers

Any type of break or lesion on the skin is a wound

Wounds occur often and they can affect anyone. Generally, regular wounds heal quickly. Ulcers, just as chronic wounds, are injuries, wounds or sores that do not heal in 30 days due to the fact that the normal mechanisms of repair are altered. Ulcers occur mostly in elderly people or patients with some co-morbidity.

In 2000, in the United States, 3.7 million people suffered from lower extremity chronic ulcers and the cost of treating them exceeded 10 billion dollars. The application of the hyperbaric oxygen therapy (HBOT), as part of the integral treatment of chronic wounds, avoids amputations of limbs, shortens the hospital stay and assists in the health and overall recovery of the patients.

Why Some Ulcers Do Not Heal?

Wounds can be limited to the superficial layer of the skin, but sometimes extend into the deeper tissues that serve as support to the skin. The treatment of a wound depends on its depth and size, and how long it has been present. Wounds that do not heal within two or three months are considered chronic, and over time their healing gets more and more difficult. The famous ancient Greek physician

Hippocrates said: "Healing is a matter of time, but it is also a matter of opportunity." If the ulcer becomes chronic, the opportunity for healing it diminishes.

The process of healing requires energy. This energy is produced in each cell with the help of oxygen which is transported through the bloodstream. Oxygen crosses the wall of the tiny blood vessels called capillaries and enters into the tissues. Nerves throughout the skin are very important in treatment: they guide this process like an orchestra conductor. These nerves are altered in patients who suffer diabetes, have had poliomyelitis or a stroke or other neurological diseases.

Lack of circulation causes poor oxygen supply to the tissues, which is common in patients with diabetes or with arterial insufficiency in the legs. The cells feel suffocated and are incapable of growing and reproducing themselves, something that is essential for healing.

With insufficient oxygen around the wound, an infection can take place and the treatment process slows down.

In the past, the goal of treatment was simply to protect the wound with a bandage, and the reconstruction of the affected structures was left to Nature.

Nowadays, medical practice provides factors lacking in the human body: such as insulin, oxygen and other. Modern therapies: hyperbaric chambers, negative pressure pumps, vacuum dressings, wound care products with growth factors, etc., create favorable conditions for enhanced wound healing. In these conditions the special attention is paid to providing oxygen to the tissues.

Role of Oxygen in the Treatment of Wounds

Hyperbaric oxygen turns out to be more than fresh air for the suffocated cell.

If oxygen is available, tissue cells can produce the energy, necessary for them to survive, multiply, and grow; closing the negative space created by the ulcer

Oxygen stimulates the growth of new blood vessels and increases the activity of cells forming collagen, the basic substance of healing

- Atoms of oxygen enter like a structural element into the collagen molecule

It is common knowledge that a thoroughbred horse that has suffered a severe fracture in a leg is sacrificed. Nevertheless, at the veterinary center of the San Isidro race track in suburban Buenos Aires, Argentina, these cases are treated successfully in a special hyperbaric chamber for horses. Veterinarian Federico Oyuela showed us the x-ray of an animal's leg with an open fracture that managed to heal after a series of treatments in the hyperbaric chamber. Skeptics that attribute the beneficial effects of the hyperbaric chamber to human psychology, as if this treatment could act as placebo, may change their minds after seeing its effects on animals.

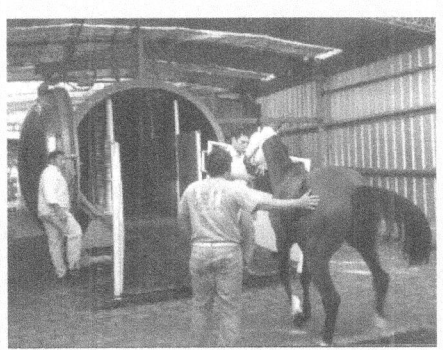

Arabian horse is introduced into the hyperbaric chamber to treat head trauma.

The veterinarian in charge of the hyperbaric chamber observes her patient.

- Oxygen promotes nerve recovery, allowing them to transmit information correctly, and thereby promote healing
- Oxygen enhances the defenses of patients against microbes because:
  1. Oxygen inhibits the growth of bacteria that do not tolerate high oxygen partial pressures (anaerobic)
  2. It increases the ability of white blood cells to destroy microorganisms by digestion, which is called "phagocytosis"
  3. Intensifies the potency of some antibiotics
- There is an important additional effect of hyperbaric oxygen in the treatment of the wounds not previously known: it increases the sensitivity of the cells to "growth factors," substances that allow the tissue to grow rapidly

So, hyperbaric oxygen plays a crucial role in wound healing.

The Hyperbaric Chamber Accelerates the Treatment of Wounds

First in observing this phenomenon were the divers of Jacques Yves Cousteau, who noticed that their wounds healed more quickly, when they lived in Jacques Cousteau's subsea habitat in the Red Sea at 10 meters below the surface.

This healing took place because at that depth they experienced twice the atmospheric pressure as on the surface. Consequently, oxygen partial pressure also rises to twice normal level and its presence in the blood increases and it saturates tissues better.

The Hyperbaric Chamber. Science, Not Miracle

Even in patients with poor circulation, the pressure in a hyperbaric chamber forces more oxygen into the tissues.

It is not necessary to live permanently in a hyperbaric chamber to accelerate the healing of wounds. It is sufficient to receive pure oxygen in a hyperbaric chamber for one hour or an hour and a half per day.

When the session is finished, extra oxygen remains in the tissues for up to four hours. This is how an additional therapeutic effect is achieved.

- When to begin treatment. The results are better when treatment begins early, because over time, tissues around the wound become fibrous, which worsen circulation and delay healing. The wound surface should contract as it heals, but the fibrous tissues prevent this and the healing process is held up.
- What treatment pressure is needed? It is generally enough with a pressure twice greater than atmospheric pressure.
- How long is each treatment? Usually one hour.
- What about frequency? It depends on the clinical evaluation of the patient: daily, every two days or twice a week
- How many sessions? In our experience, most patients need an average of 40 treatments.

Recomendations

- If during two months of standard therapy an ulcer has not healed, it is time to consult your physician and ask him about treatment with hyperbaric oxygen.
- Hyperbaric oxygen therapy is complementary factor in the treatment of wounds. Medical treatment,

surgery, application of antibiotics when necessary, counseling, and other components, should comprise the treatment process.
- Combination with other techniques makes treatment more efficient. For example, the concurrent use of hyperbaric oxygen therapy and modern dressings achieves good results.
- During the treatment the patient should avoid feeling cold, pain or stress. He or she should not smoke. All these conditions constrict blood vessels and reduce circulation. In particular, smoking one cigarette contracts the arteries for one hour. If the person has smoked five cigarettes a day, blood flow in the low extremities was reduced for five hours. Smoking a package of 20 cigarettes affects normal circulation for the period of 24 hours.

Diabetic Foot Ulcer

An attractive, good looking woman is sitting in front of me. Four days ago she was at a party. She wasn't feeling any discomfort yet in the big toe of her right foot, but a tragedy was going on. Her stocking had torn, making a running knot around the toe. When she came home and took off her shoe, her toe had turned purple.

Her toe should have been amputated and it was. And yet, the pathological process continued putting her at risk of losing her foot. Why? She is diabetic.

We started her on hyperbaric oxygen (HBO) treatment. The patient began to breathe pure oxygen while her body was in a special chamber at twice the ambient pressure. According to Henry's law of physics, the amount of gas that dissolves into a liquid is proportional to the partial pressure exerted by the gas on the liquid. So, oxygen is becoming more soluble in blood and with circulation it is delivered to the tissues in greater quantity. Cells that were starving for oxygen start to recover.

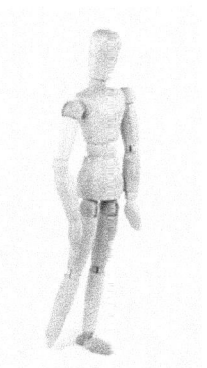

Our treatment lasted almost one month, five times a week, one hour each HBO session. First, the skin around the amputated toe acquired a normal color. Granulation tissue consisting of new blood vessels was budding on the amputation site. Gradually new skin was growing over the healing tissue. The risk of losing her foot was gone and the woman was able to return to normal life.

Blood Sugar

When explaining this disease to my patients, I liken a body to an office building, where one needs a porter named Insulin to open the doors. Let us imagine the offices as the body's cells, the corridors as arteries and people as sugar. When Insulin is present and in a good mood, there are no problems. He opens the doors and the people have free access to their offices. In this way Insulin regulates the entry of sugar into the cells. When Insulin disappears (type 1 diabetes) or is lazy (type 2 diabetes), he doesn't open the doors and the office workers cannot enter their offices, staying in the corridors, which become overcrowded. The blood of a diabetic patient without insulin contains more sugar than necessary while the cells get less sugar than necessary. There are many workers in the hallways and few in their offices.

Problems of Sugar Excess

A condition in which an excessive amount of sugar or glucose circulates in the blood is called hyperglycemia or high blood sugar. Chronic hyperglycemia at levels slightly above normal can produce a variety of serious complications, damaging kidneys, nerves, arteries, retina, etc. Hyperglycemia induces a chain of chemical reactions, whose prod-

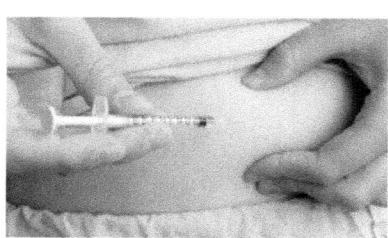

ucts modify the state of muscles, tendons, ligaments and fascias, or connective tissue that surrounds muscles, group of muscles, blood vessels and nerves, getting all of them "glycated" and therefore sticky as an old rubber.

If a non diabetic sprains his or her ankle, black and blue marks or bruises called hematoma appear, which are progressively reabsorbed by the body. In a diabetic patient in the same situation, the injury is always greater: hematoma can be accompanied by tissue necrosis because of the stickiness of glycated connective tissue.

> HBOT has been shown to reduce amputation rates in a prospective, randomized controlled clinical trial when compared to standard therapy that included revascularization, debridement, treatment of infection and glycemic control

Once necrosis appears, for example in a toe, white blood cells amass trying to isolate the affected area. Blood flow is obstructed and the area swells. Blood circulation progressively diminishes, and so more and more tissue is dying or getting necrotized.

The excess glucose in the blood also produces another disorder: nerve damage. It is called diabetic neuropathy. This phenomenon interferes with the transmission of messages between the brain and other body parts. Without any real reason the patient can feel pain, tingling, burning or, on the contrary, loss of feeling— numbness—in hands and feet. This was the case of our patient with the stocking problem: she didn't feel pain. Because of the neuropathy the sweat glands in the skin don't

> **When to use HBOT**
> - If wound is not progressing toward healing in 4-week standard therapy, then HBOT should be considered
> - All previous treatments should continue to be utilized

function properly, so skin turns dry and easy to break. The loss of nervous control may cause muscle weakness and modify reflexes, changing the way a person walks. This produces foot deformities, for example, hammertoes, which increase local pressure in the toes, causing blisters and sores to appear.

Insulin Resistance

Many patients with type 2 diabetes have insulin resistance. This means that the normal mechanism of interaction of insulin with the cells is broken. In our example, when the porter named Insulin opens the door of the offices, it would be as if Insulin is carrying keys that do not match the keyholes. And so, in an effort to keep blood sugar at the normal level the pancreas discharges more and more insulin.

Gradually, the cells that produce insulin in the pancreas become exhausted and finally the number of these cells also diminishes. And insulin resistance is also associated with a greater proportion of "bad" cholesterol and lower levels of "good" cholesterol in the blood. That is why plaques of cholesterol are deposited in the walls of arteries. Cholesterol plaques cause hardening of arterial walls and narrowing of the inner channel of the artery, hindering blood flow. This is the reason for blood vessel insufficiency in the lower limbs. This impairment to the blood vessels is called "vasculopathy" or "angiopathy".

How Does Hyperbaric Oxygen Therapy Act?

It increases the amount of dissolved oxygen in the blood, so this gas spreads deeper into the tissues making their recovery possible.

Swelling is diminished. The swelling (edema) which appears around the damaged zone is harmful. It is like a water bag that tightens the arteries. Because of diabetes, blood flow in the lower limb arteries is reduced by the plaques in the vessels walls, but when swelling appears, the blood flow decreases even more. A vicious cycle begins, a complex series of events that reinforces itself through a feedback loop toward greater instability: reduced circulation –edema– circulation is reduced even more, etc. But hyperbaric oxygen treatment breaks this vicious cycle and reduces the edema.

New blood vessels grow. Oxygen stimulates the synthesis of substances that are the basis of our flesh and skin, so the defect, created by the ulcer, is covered with new tissue. The main substance is a protein called collagen. For its production a certain quantity of molecular oxygen is required. With lack of oxygen collagen weakens, and ulcers that seemed to be healed open again.

The same substance –collagen– is needed to form new blood vessels or capillaries. When they grow sufficiently, the problem of diabetic foot ulcer can finally be resolved. The new capillaries improve

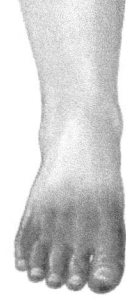

oxygen and nutrients supply to the tissues. Italian physicians measured the amount of oxygen in the feet of their patients using transcutaneous sensors before and after the hyperbaric chamber treatment. Before the treatment patients had levels of oxygen beneath the critical (so ulcers appeared) and after 30 or 40 HBO applications this level grew reaching normal values, thus, not only foot ulcers were cured, but the risk of future injury decreased significantly.

Recovery of resistance to infection. The white cells capacity to kill bacteria that invade wounds decreases with the lack of oxygen. Hyperbaric oxygen treatment clearly increases this capacity and also directly enhances the effect of some antibiotics.

Blood glucose becomes more stable. When HBO is added to the treatment protocol, there is an improvement in blood glucose control. The levels of blood sugar become more stable and the patient needs less insulin or oral hypoglycemic agents.

Factors regulating a variety of cellular processes increase. In the process of healing the key position belongs to substances called "growth factors". They promote the growth, proliferation and maturation of cells. Growth factors provide signals to neighboring cells on what to do in order to cover the ulcer bed. HBO multiplies the number of receptors on cell membranes that capture growth factors, stimulating wound healing.

When HBO Treatment Should Begin?

Small injuries as bruises and sores generally heal by their own with minimal standard therapy. Deep ulcers that invade bone, tendons, joints and fascias require the inclusion of HBO in the treatment, which comprises also diabetes medical treatment, blood glucose control, and in cases of severe arterial insufficiency in the limbs, surgical revascularization for the restoration of blood supply.

There are two revascularization procedures: bypass, consisting in rerouting the blood flow through another vessel to avoid the obstructed portion of the artery; and angioplasty, which widens narrowed or blocked blood vessels by means of a balloon tipped-catheter. Both approaches restore blood circulation and accelerate wound healing. The results depend on where the blockage was and on how much blockage a patient has in others arteries. In many cases HBO application is useful after revascularization. In patients that for any reason cannot be subjected to surgical revascularization, the hyperbaric chamber is the last recourse before limb amputation.

How Many HBO Sessions are Needed and How Long is Each Treatment?

The quantity of HBO applications vary from one patient to another, there are not two persons with the same clinical picture. According to our clinical experience, the mean is about 40 HBO sessions. Generally, the sessions last one hour, and in case of severe infection, 90 minutes.

How Efficient is this Treatment?

Jorge, a young man, diabetic from childhood, injured a big toe. The wound became severely infected and foot amputation seemed inevitable. He received 15 sessions of hyperbaric oxygen treatment and the wound improved so obviously that the recommendation of foot amputation was changed to toe amputation. After another 15 HBO applications the toe was also saved. Two years later Jorge suffered another foot injury. This time he came up right away to our Hyperbaric Center. In ten HBO sessions he was cured. Sometimes he comes to say hello. On his last visit we shared his joy at having graduated as a psychologist from the Buenos Aires State University.

The hyperbaric oxygen treatment is effective only if patient is compliant. If he or she ignores diet, medication, local wound treatment and physical exercise, treatment will result in low efficiency.

We have treated hundreds of patients with diabetic foot ulcers with 70-80% cured or improved so as to receive a skin graft if the injury was too large to wait for natural healing. In many cases, amputations were avoided or were less than anticipated, for example, amputating a toe instead of the foot, or a foot instead of a leg.

Our results coincide with data published in the peer-reviewed journals. Physicians from Italy, France, USA and Sweden report many cases of diabetic foot ulcers when thanks to HBO application limbs were saved or it was possible to reduce the amputation level and help patient to walk again. The worldwide experience of the last 30 years of HBO application in diabetic foot ulcers is enormous. In the Web there are many scientific papers that justify the use of HBO in such cases. In Table 1 and Table 2 we show a selection of international data.

Evidence Based Medicine and HBO in Diabetic Foot Ulcer Treatment

Over the last four decades there has been a six-fold increase in diabetes mellitus in the United States. Lower extremity amputations among the diabetic people increased from 67,000 in 1994 to 140,000 in 2000. The economic and social burden of diabetic foot ulcers and their complications are huge.

Amputations		
Study	With HBO	Without HBO
Oriani 1990 (80)	5%	33%
Doctor 1992 (30)	13%	47%
Faglia 1996 (68)	9%	33%
Kalani 2002 (17)	12%	33%

Table 1. Amputations in patients treated with and without HBO. In parenthesis the number of patients included in the study..

	Healed	
	With HBO	Without HBO
Baroni 1987 (28)	88%	10%
Oriani 1990 (80)	95%	67%
Stone 1995 (469)	78%	53%
Zamboni 1997 (10)	80%	20%
Abidia 2001 (18)	68%	29%
Kalani 2002 (17)	76%	48%

Table 2. Percentage of patients healed with and without HBO. The scientific level of cited studies is consistent with evidence based medicine and should be taken into account in health care policy decisions.

Annual revision of evidence based medicine gives physicians the current and most effective tools to save limbs and lives. The leader in this field, Georgetown University Hospital, has developed the Diabetic Limb Salvage program, which comprises a team approach to treatment, integrating vascular, plastic, and orthopedic surgery, along with basic and advanced diabetes treatment and modern wound healing technology. Annually, a Diabetic Limb Salvage conference is held, which works out consensus recommendations on the standard care of diabetic foot ulcers. The 2010 conference asserted that diabetic limb salvage involves a team effort. Any missing link in the chain of treatment increases the likelihood of amputation. And hyperbaric oxygen treatment is one of these links.

Physicians Knowledge and Attitude towards HBO

How are diabetic foot ulcers managed in practice? Do all patients who need this treatment have access to it? Are there barriers to the use of HBOT?

In many occasions speaking with patients and their families about how to get a referral to a hyperbaric medicine center, I have heard that doctor "X" or doctor "Y" does not believe in hyperbaric therapy. First, it is not a religion, so one doesn't need to have faith in a method of treatment as it is medical science. Second, is this happening only in Argentina? Do other doctors refuse HBO treatment? It was very interesting for me to find a scientific study about this problem.

A group of Canadian and American physicians explored physicians' knowledge of hyperbaric medicine and their attitude towards HBO therapy. In 2006 they made a survey at a primary care medicine conference. Less than 10% of doctors had good knowledge of HBOT, but 57% had a good attitude toward HBOT. Good knowledge on the subject was common in physicians in their forties, with 20 years of practice and who already had referred patients for treatment.

The researchers concluded that primary care physicians have underdeveloped knowledge of HBOT, but their generally positive attitudes towards its use suggest that they might be receptive to educational interventions. So, the solution is educating both physicians and patients about HBOT. This education is cost-effective, and might encourage future use of HBO.

Patients Knowledge and Attitude towards HBO

What about patients? What do they think about treatment in hyperbaric chamber? Let us consider a study from Sweden. How diabetic patients with limb-threatening foot lesions perceive and evaluate treatment with hyperbaric oxygen? Patients saw HBO treatment as part of a well-functioning health-care service. They accepted this high-technology environment in both technical aspect and relation with staff.

Our Advice for Diabetic Patients

- After reading this book you have some basic knowledge about HBO
- If you have a wound in your foot that is not cured in 30 days, ask your physician about adding HBO to the standard therapy
- If a recalcitrant osteomyelitis or progressive necrotizing infection takes place, HBO treatment should be considered even within four weeks of waiting for the outcome of standard treatment

> 70-80% of patients with diabetic foot ulcers treated with hyperbaric oxygen are cured or improved, amputations are avoided or are more conservative than anticipated, for example, amputating a toe instead of the foot, or a foot instead of a leg.

Gas Gangrene and Others Infections

Bacteria that cause infections (called pathogenic bacteria) are classified into two groups: aerobic or aerobe bacteria that survive and grow in an oxygenated environment, and anaerobic bacteria or anaerobe that do not require oxygen for growth and may even die if oxygen is present. The anaerobes live generally in body parts poor in oxygen, for example, in the digestive tract, mostly in colon and in feces; in the vagina; in the plaque beneath the gums, etc. From these places, bacteria can attack any part of the body. If their growth gets out of control it can evolve to a terrible infection, which if untreated may cause severe illness, even death. In the environment anaerobic bacteria can survive in the form of spores. The spores permit their living in a dormant state until they are exposed to favorable conditions, for

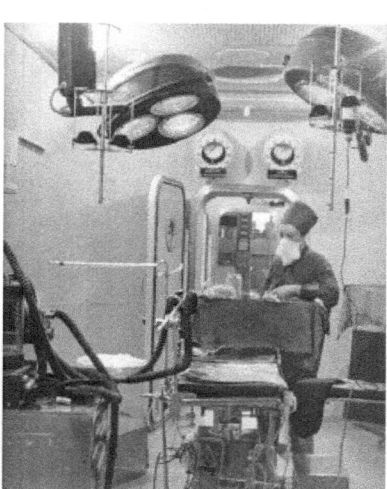

Operating room within a hyperbaric chamber at the Moscow Barocenter.
Courtesy of Professor
S.N. Efuni, M.D., Ph.D.

example, entering human organism during trauma.

Aerobic bacteria abound in the environment, also in human skin and mucosa. Our body possesses various mechanisms for fighting microorganisms, one is called phagocytosis. It consists of the engulfing and digesting of intruders by white blood cells. In traumatized or infected (septic) tissue the presence of oxygen decreases, what favors infection.

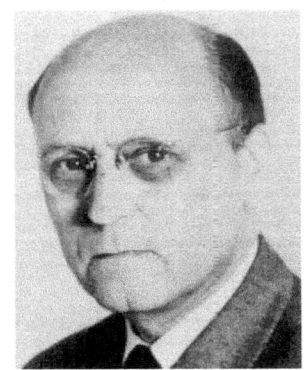

Ite Boerema, the father of modern hyperbaric medicine

Breathing oxygen in a hyperbaric chamber greatly enhances its solubility in blood compared to normal air breathing. With HBO the oxygen partial pressure in tissues reaches levels at which anaerobic bacteria cannot survive.

At the same time, when a patient is receiving hyperbaric oxygen treatment, white blood cells are stimulated, so they engulf and digest bacteria more efficiently. Besides, it is ascertained that hyperbaric oxygen also increases the bactericidal capacity of some antibiotics.

Gas Gangrene

On October 25th of 1960 the first patient with gas gangrene was treated in a hyperbaric chamber. The idea for the treatment, and its successful execution, belong to the famous Dutch physician Dr. Ite Boerema from Wilhelmina Gasthius Hospital, in Amsterdam.

Today, it is a worldwide accepted method of gas gangrene treatment. Although this infection was considered

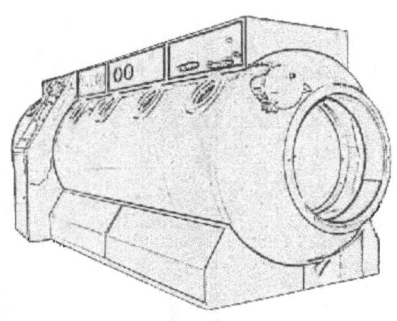

Multiple seat chamber at the Buenos Aires Hyperbaric Medicine Center.

as a war disease, it is still presenting today in everyday life.

Approximately 1,000 to 3,000 cases of clostridial gas gangrene are reported per year in U.S. Why?

The number of patients with a debilitated immune system is growing. These patients are survivors from diseases considered fatal in the past, for example, malignant tumors and diabetes, as well as patients with organ transplants and on dialysis. This group of patients is prone to developing infections. Approximately 80% of patients with non traumatic gas gangrene have an overt or occult malignancy. The probability of infections also increases by the application of new therapeutic methods with catheters and others devices introduced into the body.

Gas gangrene is a highly lethal infection caused by toxin and gas-generating bacteria of Clostridium species. It is also called clostridial myonecrosis because of producing necrosis of soft tissue and muscles. Two conditions should coexist for developing this infection: bacterial invasion into the tissues and low oxygen tension for microorganism proliferation.

These bacteria are very violent, producing up to 20 different toxins that turn out to be tissue-destructive. The most harmful is phospholipase C, typified as "Alfa"-toxin that attacks cell membranes and in a short time destroys soft tissues and red blood cells. It affects the cardiac function and stimulates thrombus formation. Theta toxin

> **Hyperbaric oxygen in gas gangrene and soft tissue necrotizing infection:**
> - Is life-saving
> - Is limb and tissue-saving

causes hemolysis or the breakdown of red blood cells, white blood cells degeneration, and destruction of polymorphonuclear cells, the main protagonists of phagocytosis or defense. Kappa toxin is a collagenase that destroys connective tissue, facilitating the rapid spread of necrosis. These effects may explain the relatively minor host inflammatory response and rapid infection propagation. To stop toxin production high oxygen partial pressure is necessary, which could be achieved only in hyperbaric chamber.

A kind of vicious cycle is formed: the bacteria destroy tissues and erythrocytes, dead masses appear in an environment poor of oxygen, creating favorable conditions to enhance bacterial growth.

The gas produced by bacteria causes swelling and "crepitation" of tissues: touching the affected zone, one feels it "crackle", the spreading of this zone is very rapid and can be directly observed. Death can arise in 24 hours.

Treatment of Gas Gangrene

A three-pronged approach forms the basis of gas gangrene treatment: antibiotics, surgery and HBO. Hyperbaric oxygen combines with all other treatments and should be applied as soon as possible.

During hyperbaric therapy, a patient can receive endovenous antibiotics and other life saving solutions. The final results depend on the combination of these three basic weapons against the disease. Dr. Desola Alá from Barcelona, Spain, an outstanding specialist in hyperbaric medicine, proposes the following formula of the success:

$$\frac{A \times S \times O}{t}$$

where
A = Antibiotics
S = Surgery
O = Hyperbaric Oxygen
t = time between the beginning of the disease and the commencement of an integrated treatment.

The numerator is a product. If just one of the three factors is very small the final result will be deplorable even if the others two measures are carried to the extreme. On other hand, when the denominator is large (too much time elapsing before applying treatment) the results will be poor.

The hyperbaric chamber doesn't replace any classic method of gas gangrene treatment, it only modifies surgery management.

In the case of a patient treated in hyperbaric chamber, initial surgery can be restricted to opening the wound and eliminating only obviously necrotic tissues avoiding radical amputations. The patient should receive three hyperbaric treatments within the first 24 hours.

Then the wound is reviewed and decisions are made about amputation. In many clinical cases it is feasible to avoid (or make minor) limb amputation, achieving a better quality of life for the patient. Later, HBO sessions are conducted once or twice a day. Generally, no more than 10 treatments are needed.

The hyperbaric chamber doesn't modify antibiotic treatment.

Fabio, 20, suffered gas gangrene after a car accident. After classic combination of antibiotics and surgery at the hospital he was rushed to our clinic. The infection was propagating from the shoulder to the thorax. This zone was reddish and crepitated to the touch.

Endovenous antibiotics were continued while in chamber. Hyperbaric oxygen sessions (five in total) and surgery followed during three days. The zone of crepitation disappeared, the wound cleaned and the process of healing began, which was completed some weeks later.

Treatment Results

Different authors from different countries have reported between 30 and 60% of mortality if gas gangrene is properly treated. If untreated, the disease is 100% fatal.

Non traumatic origin infections with abdomen involvement cause a mortality rate of 80-100%.

Doctor Desola Alá from Barcelona found that the HBO application reduces mortality to 20-40% in cases of abdominal localization or spontaneous beginning and to 5-15% in traumatic cases. 80% of patients survived. Half of them have had a complete recovery without amputations and only in one sixth major amputations were performed.

HBO in gas gangrene

1. Stops toxin production
2. Enhances phagocytosis
3. Demarks between dead and viable tissues

Soft Tissue Necrotizing Infections

Everything that is not bone is called soft tissue: muscles, subcutaneous fat, skin, etc. The infections of soft tissue usually appear after trauma or surgery. The affected patients always have some co-morbidity, or accompanying disease or condition: diabetes, vascular insufficiency, or other issues that reduce the defense of the body and the supply of oxygen to the tissues.

These infections are named by the affected tissue and some characteristic feature of the disease: crepitant anaerobic cellulitis, progressive bacterial gangrene, necrotizing fasciitis, Fournier's gangrene and nonclostridial myonecrosis. The main therapy is surgery and antibiotics. However, the common theme in these infections is hypoxia and its consequences. Hyperbaric oxygen is a complementary therapy that may be lifesaving and cost effective, because it acts against mixed microflora.

In 1984, Dr. Bakker, Dr. Boerema's successor, reviewed almost 500 scientific papers about gas gangrene and necrotizing soft tissue infection treatment and concluded that in the hospitals where hyperbaric chambers are available, mortality and amputations rate were significantly reduced.

In a generalized infection called sepsis, hyperbaric oxygen is also recommended. In Mar del Plata, Argentina, doctors Gustavo Mauvecin and Carlos Espinosa have successful experience treating pediatric population with sepsis adding the hyperbaric chamber to the standard protocol.

The treatment protocol should be individualized for each patient according to the vital signs and general state of health.

Osteomyelitis

Osteomyelitis is a bone infection caused by bacteria and fungi. Infection may reach a bone from infected skin, muscles, chronic skin ulcer or from any part of the body, spreading to the bone through the blood. The bone may be more likely to develop the infection because of a current or past injury, trauma, or low defenses. Chronic osteomyelitis may lead to amputation more common in patients with diabetes, peripheral vascular insufficiency, or immune system disorder.

The standard treatment consists of antibiotics. Sometimes surgery is needed for removal of the affected part of the bone, and in all cases techniques for stimulating the growth of new bone are required. HBO stimulates bone regeneration, which enhances the therapeutic results notably. The protocol includes 40-60 HBO sessions.

Severe trauma

Trauma has been frequent in the history of mankind. Earthquakes, building collapses, military conflicts and wars, industry disasters and traffic accidents continuously generate severe injuries. The worldwide number of seriously injured patients is growing every year. If it were a disease it would have reached epidemic proportions. Trauma is the third leading cause of death in the United States, after cardiovascular diseases and cancer, and it is the first leading cause of death for all people under the age of 44.

When a body part is squeezed between heavy objects, this severe trauma is called crush syndrome. Crush injuries can result in bleeding, bruising, broken bones, open

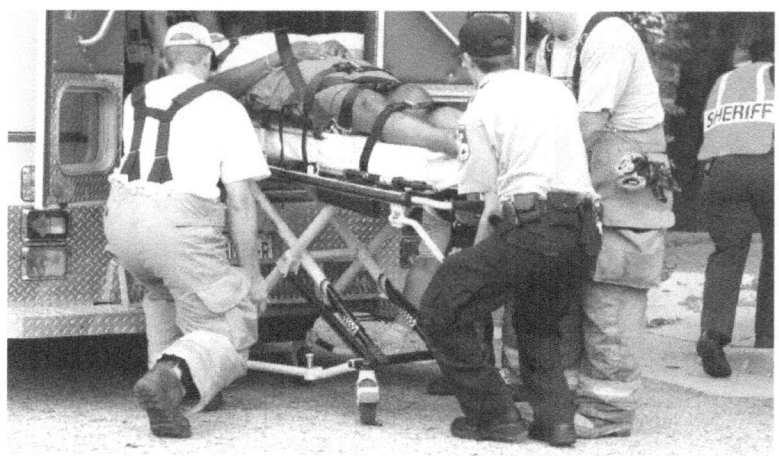

wounds and other conditions. The crushed tissues die, so toxic substances and waste products are released into circulation, causing an inflammatory response by the body.

The most important characteristic of this syndrome is blood circulation stoppage because blood vessels are affected. This condition is called acute traumatic ischemia. Ischemia is lack of blood supply. The ischemic tissues are short of oxygen and pass through certain typical stages before death. By not producing energy, cells lose control of their membranes, and the intracellular liquid leaks into the intercellular space causing swelling (edema), which in turn worsens the poor local circulation. It is as if the arteries were squeezed by a bag of water, impairing blood flow already affected by trauma. The increased liquid between cells results in the onset of compartment syndrome or compression of nerves, blood vessels, and muscles inside compartments (closed spaces surrounded by connective tissue) in the limbs. The pressure of this fluid hinders blood flow to the point of complete obstruction, causing ischemia.

Acute traumatic ischemia, severe in essence, also promotes the development of infections. There are always

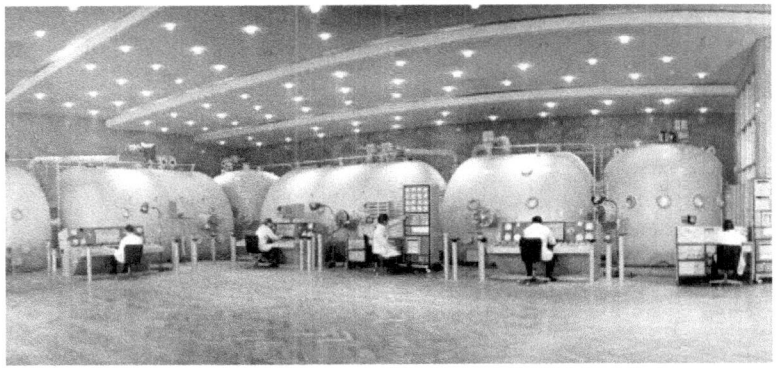

The Hyperbaric Medicine Institute named Barocenter in Moscow constructed in 1974. Courtesy of Professor S.N. Yefuni, M.D., Ph.D.

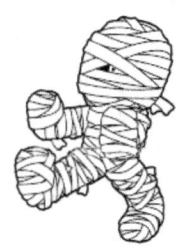

microorganisms on the skin, in the mouth, in the bowels, in the vagina and at the tip of the urethra. In a healthy person they are harmless. But when defenses lessen, these microorganisms are activated; they become virulent, causing infection from severe to mortal. The lack of oxygen means the death sentence for tissues. The dead or necrotic tissue is a breeding ground for microorganisms. When blood supply is insufficient, microbes proliferate without control and antibiotics do not reach the areas that need them. In these circumstances white blood cells lose their ability to destroy bacteria and fungi by phagocytosis. When the amount of oxygen in the tissues is high, oxygen attacks the microorganisms and puts an end to their uncontrolled growth. Therefore, there is a clear need of urgent hyperbaric oxygen (HBO) treatment in crush injuries.

HBO therapy should accompany reparative and orthopedic surgery in acute traumatic ischemia. Once the initial urgency has passed, HBO should be continued because wounds need additional oxygen for collagen production, for angiogenesis (new blood vessels formation) and for tissues repair. If oxygen is lacking, all these processes are held back.

Hyperbaric Oxygen in Acute Traumatic Ischemia

The first effect is tissue oxygenation. While a patient is receiving treatment in a hyperbaric chamber, a greater quantity of oxygen is dissolved in his or her blood reaching cells beyond the capillaries, and in many clinical cases saving these deep tissues.

The second effect is vasoconstriction or a slight constriction of the arteries, by which swelling or edema is diminished. With vasoconstriction arterial blood flow is reduced. As the venous return isn't modified, the amount of liquid entering a certain area is less than the amount going out, and therefore swelling is reduced. Although less blood is circulating, more oxygen is supplied to the tissues. The edema in patients treated with hyperbaric oxygen disappears 5-7 days earlier than in patients not treated in hyperbaric chamber.

> **Hyperbaric oxygen therapy in acute traumatic ischemia:**
>
> - less mortality
> - less limb amputations
> - complete recovery in greater proportion of patients
> - less infectious complications
> - shorter hospital stay
> - shorter recovery period

The third beneficial effect of hyperbaric chamber in severe trauma is infection control. Oxygen directly kills anaerobic microbes and enhances the power of some antibiotics. In addition, in the presence of high partial pressure of oxygen white blood cells recover their ability to kill microorganisms by phagocytosis.

The tissues of an injured patient could be classified in three categories:

1. healthy or minimally damaged
2. severely damaged, and
3. nonviable

The first two groups are favored by the HBO treatment: their viability increases and infection is controlled or prevented. The nonviable tissue could not be resuscitated, but hyperbaric oxygen prevents the expansion of infection and delineates the border between viable and nonviable tissues. The surgeon sees what parts of the limbs are recoverable and which can not be rescued, thus eliminating only necrotic tissue and avoiding a greater amputation.

Treatment Outcomes

In 1981, Dr. Michael Strauss from Long Beach, CA, analyzed 700 cases of acute traumatic ischemia published in papers by different authors. There was an obvious benefit for patients because the treatment with hyperbaric oxygen helped to avoid many amputations. In 1987, a group of Israeli physicians showed that the use of hyperbaric chamber prevented amputation in 75% of patients with impaired circulation in the limbs. The *Journal of Trauma* published in 1996 a study with a high scientific level by Dr. Bouachour and his colleagues in France, which showed the benefit of using hyperbaric oxygen in crush injuries.

Patient with acute traumatic ischemia in the right lower limb with indication of amputation because the gunshot had breached his artery. Surgery combined with HBO saved his leg.

In this study 36 patients with crush injuries were divided in blind random fashion into two groups. The two groups were similar in terms of age, risk factors, type or location of vascular injuries, neurologic injuries and fractures. Both groups received the same standard therapy: procedures and timing of surgery, antibiotics, wound dressings, etc. But one group from the first 24 hours after evaluation and the initial surgery received HBO at 2.5 atmosphere absolute (ATA) for 90 minutes, twice daily, over 6 days, total 12 sessions. The second group was treated with the same frequency with placebo (session with air practically at normal pressure. This was the one and only difference between these groups. So the difference in clinical outcome was determined only by HBO treatment.

Complete healing was obtained for 17 patients in the HBO group (94%) vs. 10 patients in the placebo group (56%). New surgical procedures (such as skin flaps and grafts, vascular surgery, or even amputation) were performed on one patient (1%) in the HBO group vs. six patients (33.3%) in the placebo group.

In Buenos Aires we have applied hyperbaric oxygen in the treatment of patients with a great loss of tissues in the limbs (skin, subcutaneous fat tissue, muscles and sometimes bone). The hyperbaric oxygen sessions reduced amputations and complications from infections.

> In 2006, the United States Congress approved a budget of $2million for the purchase, installation and use of two hyperbaric chambers to treat soldiers wounded in Iraq and Afghanistan.
>
> Previously, the Medical Center of the Air Force in that country had confirmed the benefits of hyperbaric oxygen therapy for severe injuries.

The hospital stay was shorter and the quality of life after discharge better.

Hyperbaric oxygen treatment in patients with acute traumatic ischemia should begin as early as possible.

If the surgery is delayed, the patient should start treatment in the chamber. Within the first 48 to 72 hours HBO is recommended thrice daily, then, for the next 48 hours twice daily, and finally, once a day for 48-72 hours, for a total of 16 sessions in 8 days. During this time tissues that suffered a lack of oxygen get to recover. If skin grafts and flaps are applied and they become compromised, then treatment should be continued twice a day for two additional weeks to enhance the growth of new capillaries. If the case is complicated by osteomyelitis we recommend using up to 60 sessions of hyperbaric chamber.

Firearm Wounds

The experience of military physicians in Croatia in the early 1990s showed that when surgery was combined with hyperbaric oxygen, 189 war victims with acute traumatic ischemia in the extremities had a good outcome.

In our Medical Center we have treated patients with limb arteries affected by gunshot wounds. This has helped surgeons to save those limbs.

Prevention of Infections

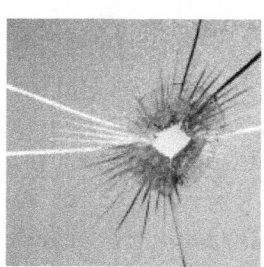

The N.V. Sklifosovsky Emergency Medicine Research Institute in Moscow (former Soviet Union) had an excellent hyperbaric medicine department that used HBO as part of its routine protocol in many difficult trauma cases. Isakov, Atroshchenko and Grigoriev published in 1980 their experiences in the treatment of patients with open fractures. In an open fracture the bone and the skin are broken; therefore there is a high risk of infection. These patients received HBO from the first 48 hours after trauma twice a day for a total of 10 sessions. The outcome of this group of patients was excellent. The infectious complication were 2.4 times less in patients treated with hyperbaric oxygen in comparison with another group of patients that suffered the same fractures but were not treated in a hyperbaric chamber.

Post Traumatic Cerebral Edema

Craneoencephalic trauma is one of the most common causes of hospitalization in emergency care units, and 50% of trauma-related deaths result from this type of injury. Lack of oxygen in the brain (cerebral hypoxia) was observed in 91% of fatal head injuries. Hypoxia is the main reason why some patients remain in a vegetative state or suffer permanent neurologic damage. In these cases it is helpful to use the hyperbaric chamber.

In response to head trauma, swelling occurs in the brain around the injured area. After a severe head injury this swelling or edema might extend to the entire brain. The brain's volume tends to increase because of the leaking of liquid from cerebral capillaries. Since the skull is a rigid structure, it doesn't allow for the enlargement of the brain. Thus, intracranial pressure rises, damaging the central nervous system by compression of cerebral structures, among them some important areas that control vital body functions such as circulation and respiration. The compression causes a decrease in blood flow and oxygen supply to the brain that in turn causes more swelling. As an additional reduction in blood flow occurs, the hypoxia or lack of oxygen in the brain worsens.

Treatment of brain swelling is difficult. Strong medications or surgery are often the only options. Surgery generally involves removing a small section of the skull in order to reduce intracranial pressure.

The overall goal of the treatment is to maintain blood flow and oxygen supply to all parts of the brain, thus minimizing the damage and increasing the probability of survival and recuperation of the patient.

HBO in Cerebral Edema Treatment

Hyperbaric oxygen therapy serves two specific important functions: increasing oxygen supply to the brain and reducing cerebral edema. How should patients be selected for this treatment? Which of them will show a better response to HBO?

To define a patient's state of consciousness, physicians use the classification named Glasgow Coma Scale, which assigns a 3 to a patient in deep coma or profound unconsciousness and 15 to fully alert person. Patients with scores 4-11 should be treated in hyperbaric chamber. Those with score 3 will not respond to treatment. Those with higher score than 11 do not need hyperbaric oxygen because they have a mild injury and would recover spontaneously.

Generally, a patient will show neurological improvement during the first few hyperbaric treatments, although its degree could vary. After each treatment, a slight regression, a kind of a small step backward in his state, may be seen as the brain re-adjusts to lower oxygen levels outside the hyperbaric chamber. However, this loss is always small, and with each consecutive session neurologic symptoms progressively disappear. HBO therapy should go on until the patient completely recovers or until there is no more improvement in his or her neurologic state with the ongoing sessions.

We have treated several patients with post traumatic cerebral edema. All were healthy before their accidents. Hyperbaric oxygen resolved the coma. All recovered consciousness. The less time passed between trauma and the beginning of HBO treatment, the faster was the retrieval of consciousness. That is why hyperbaric oxygen should be applied without delay.

The first reports about HBO application in head trauma appeared in the 1960's. Patients regained consciousness, improved mobility, speech, etc.

At the Sklifosovsky Institute in Moscow the outcome of 206 patients with craneoencephalic trauma was analyzed. Half of the patients received HBO treatment and another half not. The first group recovered consciousness more rapidly and also presented three-times less neurologic and psychiatric posttraumatic sequelae than the patients not treated in hyperbaric chamber.

In 1974, Hollbach and colleagues in Austria reported that HBO application in patients with craneoencephalic trauma diminished mortality. In the control group (without hyperbaric oxygen treatment) fatal outcomes were registered in 55% of cases and only in 6% in the group treated with hyperbaric oxygen. And, 33% of "hyperbaric" group showed a complete recovery vs. 6% in non treated group.

In Minnesota, USA, in the early 1990's Dr. G.L. Rockswold conducted an excellent clinical study on 168 patients with severe closed head injuries. The mortality of patients treated in hyperbaric chamber was of 17%, vs. 32% in a group of patients that didn't receive this treatment. And the comparison within the 80 most severely injured patients showed an even greater difference between these groups.

Conclusions:

- When hyperbaric oxygen is used on time and combined with orthopedic surgery in severe trauma, the outcome is better and the total cost of treatment is lower
- Traumatic brain injury patients treated in a hyperbaric chamber as soon as possible after the incident have better chances of survival and less neurologic and psychiatric sequelae

República de Cromagnon's Tragedy: Smoke and Toxic Gases

New Year 2005 was approaching and everyone was preparing to celebrate it. December 31st in Argentina meant an "afternoon off". Since all our patients had decided to take the day off we moved all scheduled HBO sessions to January the 2nd.

At 1:30 AM I was awakened by a phone call from an emergency physician: "Doctor, I am sending you a patient with carbon monoxide poisoning. His carboxyhemoglobin is 36%." That means that hemoglobin (the main protein of blood that carries oxygen to the tissues) is bound by carbon monoxide. This renders the involved hemoglobin unable to bind oxygen. The patient may die from asphyxia. December is a summer month in Buenos Aires, so it seemed to me very rare to receive such a patient. Usually, these poisonings occur in winter due to the malfunctioning of heaters. The emergency physician suggested that

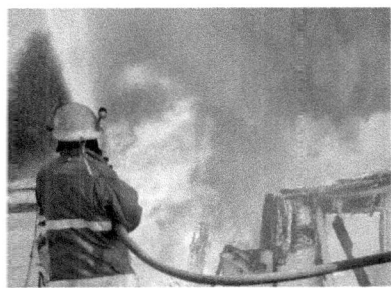

I watch the news on TV. That is how I found out about the tragedy: a fire at a nightclub (disco club) called República de Cromagnon. At that time thirty young people had already died.

Fifteen minutes later, when I was treating the patient, the TV reported that there were already 40 fatal victims. Then 50, 60... 174 young people died at the scene of the event, 726 injured persons were admitted to hospitals, and 117 to intensive care units. Later 19 persons died, raising the death toll to 193. This tragedy was the sixth on record of fire fatalities in world history, and the third if considering only those in dancing clubs.

> Breathing oxygen in a carbon monoxide poisoning saves life. The same effect of elimination of carbon monoxide from its union with hemoglobin is achieved in:
> - 320 minutes if breathing fresh air
> - 80 minutes if breathing pure oxygen under atmospheric pressure
> - 22 minutes if breathing pure oxygen in a hyperbaric chamber

I called the city medical authorities to let them know that in view of this catastrophe, patients would be attended in my clinic even if they had no health insurance.

Other patients started to arrive. We had treated 12, working from 2 AM to 6 PM. We were glad we did not have our patient's schedule workload!!!

The patients, all young, told me they had lost consciousness at some point. One girl could not control her sphincters because carbon monoxide had affected her central nervous system.

The tragedy occurred because one of the boys threw a flare that ignited the plastic decorative ceiling, and it began to fall in flames over the audience, generating toxic gases. Emergency exit doors turned out to be closed.

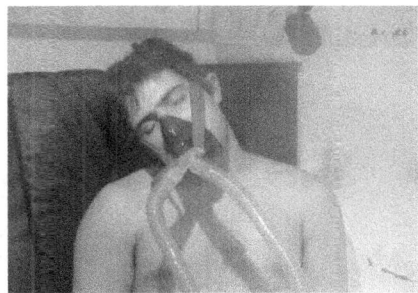

Patient from the fire of República de Cromagnon treated at our center.

How and Where Is Carbon Monoxide Produced

The chemical composition of a substance determines which gases are produced when it burns. The most common gas is carbon dioxide (CO_2). Where there is little oxygen carbon monoxide (CO) is generated. This is a very dangerous gas that is called "the silent killer" because it is invisible, colorless, odorless, and not irritating.

Sources of carbon monoxide are stoves, heaters, braziers and any faulty combustion appliances. Car exhaust gases are also highly toxic because they can contain up to 7% of carbon monoxide. In cigarette smoke, the concentration of carbon monoxide can reach 3-6%, so smokers usually have 4-5% of carboxyhemoglobin in blood. And in heavy cigarette smokers the carboxyhemoglobin level is documented above 9%.

Other Toxic Substances

The decorative ceiling of the dance club was made of polyurethane. Its combustion produced another killer par excellence: cyanide gas, one of the most rapidly acting lethal poisons known to humankind. When one more common

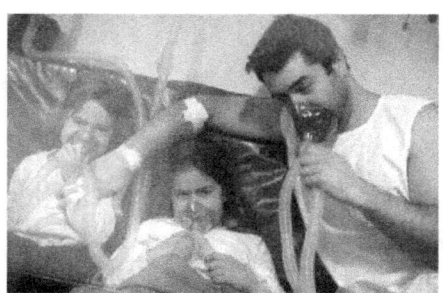

A stove in the house of this family was malfunctioning producing CO. Father and daughters lost consciousness and had to be treated in the hyperbaric chamber.

plastic - polyvinylchloride —called PVC— is burned, hydrogen chloride is formed, a very toxic and also irritating gas.

According to statistics, 50% of deaths in building fires are caused by poisoning with combustion products, not because of thermal burns.

Toxic Effects of Carbon Monoxide

Carbon monoxide avidly binds to hemoglobin, which becomes unable to carry oxygen. The capacity of carbon monoxide to combine with hemoglobin is 220 times greater than that of oxygen. This allows relatively small carbon monoxide concentrations in the environment to cause severe poisoning. Asphyxia can occur when carbon monoxide binds with only 30-40% of hemoglobin. Carbon monoxide is responsible for more than half of all fatal poisonings.

Today it is known that there are also other mechanisms of action of carbon monoxide. Besides hemoglobin binding, exogenous CO can disturb cellular metabolism because it inhibits energy production in mitochondria – the tiny power stations of the cells. In addition, it directly affects our brain tissue by destroying neuron membranes and nerve fibers. A fourth mechanism of neurological damage is produced by white blood cells that leave the bloodstream and enter the brain, inflaming it. Leukocytes enter brain tissue and create the foci of future lesions.

How to Save a Victim of CO Poisoning?

Just let him breathe oxygen. As carbon monoxide has a greater affinity for hemoglobin than oxygen, high concentrations of oxygen are needed to displace monoxide from its binding with hemoglobin.

Back in the 1950s it was established that it takes 320 minutes (more than 5 hours) to reduce by half the amount of hemoglobin affected by carbon monoxide if the patient is breathing air. This time is reduced to 80 minutes if the patient breathes oxygen by mask, and only 22 minutes if the patient breathes oxygen in a hyperbaric chamber. This is due to the fact that the body receives a greater amount of oxygen while breathing it under a pressure higher than the atmospheric one.

Oxygen at atmospheric pressure eliminates carbon monoxide from carboxyhemoglobin, but the hyperbaric oxygen also:

- recovers the cellular energy production
- protects against the destruction of cell membranes and nerve fibers
- prevents delayed neurological sequelae

Hyperbaric Oxygen in Carbon Monoxide Poisoning

The oxygen breathed in a hyperbaric chamber has a higher curative effect than when it is inhaled at atmospheric pressure. Both unlock hemoglobin, but with the hyperbaric oxygen (HBO) also the cellular energy production is recovered. In addition it protects against the destruction of cell membranes and nerve fibers, and prevents inflammation of the brain produced by white blood cells.

Monoxide Poisoning and Pregnancy

When a pregnant woman is exposed to carbon monoxide, it is transmitted to the fetus, and carboxyhemoglobin is formed in concentrations 10-15% higher than those of the mother. This difference comes from the higher affinity of fetal hemoglobin to carbon monoxide than adult hemoglobin. Oxygen given to the mother passes to the fetus through the placenta. Monoxide travels a reverse path from the fetus to the mother, who eliminates it in by the lungs. This second process is slow and takes place at a stable speed, so the fetal carboxyhemoglobin level exceeds that of the mother up to 10 hours after exposure is over.

For that reason it is common that the mother survives monoxide exposure, but not the unborn baby. There are

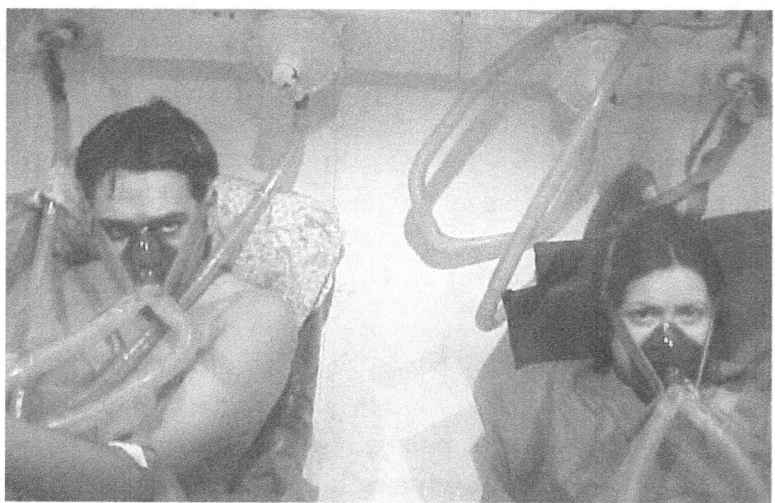

These patients, from the fire of República de Cromagnon, were treated at our center.

numerous documented cases of carbon monoxide poisoning in which the fetus dies and the mother recovers, however, if the children do survive, they often suffer from a wide range of neurological problems.

For decades, hyperbaric oxygen was contraindicated in pregnant women due to the concern that high concentration of oxygen would cause unwanted changes in fetal blood circulation. Numerous studies conducted in the former Soviet Union showed that short exposure to hyperbaric oxygen does not cause damage to fetal circulation.

Some physicians, particularly Dr. Desola Alá, in Spain, insist on treating all pregnant women after exposure to carbon monoxide, regardless of the level of carboxyhemoglobin. We also share that view.

Who Should Be Treated in the Hyperbaric Chamber?

Since 1962, severe carbon monoxide poisoning is being treated in hyperbaric chamber if the patient:

- is in a coma
- has lost consciousness even if for five minutes
- has any neurological disorders (difficulty in retaining urine or feces, blurred or double vision, etc.)
- has cardiovascular symptoms caused or aggravated by CO poisoning
- is asymptomatic with 25% or more of carboxyhemoglobin
- children in the first years of life and persons older that 65 with a lower carboxyhemoglobin level and less symptomatic
- pregnant women after carbon monoxide exposure, regardless of their carboxyhemoglobin level

> Since 1962, severe carbon monoxide poisoning is treated in hyperbaric chamber if the patient:
> - is in coma
> - has lost consciousness even if for 5 minutes
> - has neurological symptoms (difficulty in retaining urine or feces, blurred or double vision, etc.)
> - has cardiovascular symptoms caused or aggravated by carbon monoxide event
> - is asymptomatic with 25% or more of carboxyhemoglobin level
> - is a child from birth to 1 year with minimal symptoms
> - is over 65 years with low carboxyhemoglobin and with mild symptoms
> - is a pregnant woman regardless of carboxyhemoglobin level

Although children sometimes have only transient seizures of short duration, these patients should also be treated in a hyperbaric chamber.

Usually one session of HBO is enough to erase the traces of carbon monoxide from the body and prevent further complications that could affect the central nervous system.

We have a lot of experience in this field: over the last 12 years in two centers in Buenos Aires we have treated almost 2,000 patients with acute carbon monoxide poisoning. Our judgment is based on critical analysis and reflection over this unique experience.

Many patients who were exposed to CO suffer severe headaches. These headaches are localized in the front part of the skull behind the eyes, and it is believed to be related to cerebral edema. In addition, we have observed nausea, vomiting, dizziness, gastrointestinal symptoms, urinary incontinence, and rarely, skin lesions.

As a rule, all these symptoms practically disappear during the first HBO session. Patients recover normal skin tone and their headaches go away. Their appetite returns, more noticeable in children. These dramatic changes justify hyperbaric therapy for these patients. In other words, the clinical change is very positive and we have seen it in almost 2,000 patients, all of whom had been breathing normobaric oxygen before arriving at our center.

A famous intensive care physician and hyperbaric medicine specialist, Dr. Weaver from LDS Hospital in Salt Lake City, USA, showed in 2002 that 46% of patients with acute carbon monoxide poisoning not treated with hyperbaric therapy suffered nervous system complications, compared to only 25% in patients treated with hyperbaric oxygen.

Delayed Neurological Sequelae of Carbon Monoxide Poisoning

Mario, 53 years old, came to visit his father one winter Sunday in 2003. After dinner, they both went to watch television and fell asleep while a stove burnt gas with a bright orange flame, emanating carbon monoxide. Mario woke up on Tuesday breathing through an endotracheal tube. He stayed alive by a miracle. His father had passed away.

Mario recovered, but a week later worsened again as if he had a stroke. He could not eat or speak or control his sphincters. What to do? The neurologists performed a functional magnetic resonance study and found that Mario's brain, despite being severely affected, had not lost its structure completely. So, they tried to save him with the help of hyperbaric oxygen therapy. Slowly but steadily, the patient began to improve. A complete recovery was achieved after 35 sessions.

The results were so successful that Mario went back to work as a systems analyst. "Without the hyperbaric chamber I would have ended up in a vegetative state", he says. What Mario suffered is known as "late sequelae of carbon monoxide poisoning "or "delayed neurological syndrome", which means decay after a period of seeming normality. These cases usually occur between 3rd and 40th days after an apparent recovery.

The consequences can range from headache to a vegetative state. Usually mild disorders resolve spontaneously, but severe ones remain.

Aitor, 11, was found in the bathroom unconscious. After mouth-to-mouth resuscitation his father took him to the hospital where carbon monoxide poisoning was diagnosed and treatment commenced. The boy recovered with the application of oxygen by mask. He returned home and everything seemed normal. But on the fourth day he became irritable and developed a headache so strong that he was admitted back into the hospital. His condition continued to worsen and on the fifth day after the accident he was blind and in a coma. At that time he was flown to Buenos Aires by air ambulance and taken to the hyperbaric chamber. After seven HBO treatments Aitor regained consciousness, vision, mental ability and movement. Little by little he returned to normal life, but he is kept on the anticonvulsive medication, because the foci of lesions in his brain persist. Now he is 19. Every time the family is visiting Buenos Aires they come by to say hello.

Dito, 58 years old, fell into a coma after carbon monoxide exposure. The next three days he lived connected to a respirator. He recovered, but two weeks later the headaches began. The brain MRI found the typical monoxide poisoning abnormalities.

Three weeks later headaches continued. The man seemed to be normal but apathetic, unwilling to do anything. The neurologist noted that the patient walked unsteadily. The assessment of cognitive function showed that he could not solve problems, could not calculate, he spoke slowly and his voice sounded robotic. With great effort he could memorize a list of things, but getting a second list forgot the first one. He could not remember events of his life and did not recognize some family pictures. He was practically, unable to work. Walking in the street was dangerous to him, because he had to give full attention to the act of walking itself, and not to the traffic.

Hyperbaric oxygen therapy was indicated. After 20 sessions he had recovered almost completely and returned to his normal life.

Once I received a sad message from one patient. Fifteen years ago she suffered acute carbon monoxide poisoning and was treated with normobaric oxygen. She recovered, but a month after the incident she developed severe Parkinson syndrome, which wasn't linked to the previous monoxide poisoning but treated as a standard Parkinson's syndrome. Now, at the age of 45, she is a disabled person. Her story would be different had she been treated at that time in a hyperbaric chamber.

This syndrome should not be disregarded and the symptoms should not be attributed to another disease

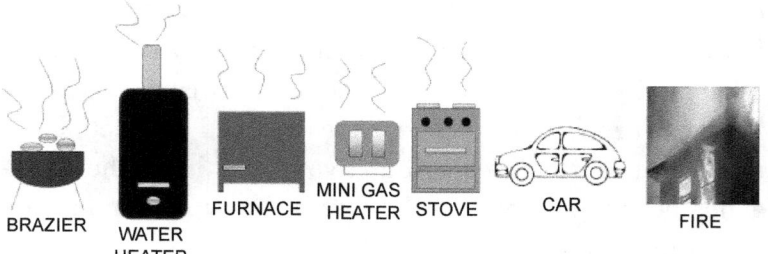

Equipment must be in good
technical condition and meet safety standards.

and treated incorrectly. That is why we instruct all our patients after an acute CO poisoning, to seek medical help at the first sign of neurological impairment or any behavior alteration within 45 days after the event. The patient should be examined by a clinician and a neurologist. In all doubtful cases, neurologic imaging should be done and the decision about applying HBO made.

Hyperbaric Oxygen in Cyanide Gas Poisoning

The cyanide gas is another hazardous substance generated by fires. The patient dies due to lack of cellular energy production. Standard therapy for this poisoning consists of 100% oxygen and antidotes. The antidotes for cyanide gas produce methemoglobin, necessary for detoxification, but unable to carry oxygen.

The blood of patients exposed simultaneously to carbon monoxide and cyanide gas contains both carboxyhemoglobin and methemoglobin. The first is produced by contact with carbon monoxide, and the second by cyanide poisoning therapy. As blood is unable to carry oxygen the application of hyperbaric oxygen therapy presents a double benefit for these patients.

The Smoke Inhalation Injury

Irritation from smoke inhalation can lead to a sequence of conditions: acute respiratory failure, pulmonary edema and bronchopneumonia.

When hyperbaric oxygen therapy was used in victims of fire to treat thermal burns, physicians noticed that in these patients pulmonary disorders also decreased.

Today we know the mechanisms by which hyperbaric oxygen therapy reduces lung injury after smoke inhalation. The time between exposure to smoke and the onset of this therapy should not exceed 12 hours, so called "the time window" before pulmonary edema and inflammation develop and HBO will become useless.

Is This Pathology Important Only in Argentina?

There are 50,000 annual visits to emergency departments in U.S. due to CO poisoning. Treated with time the vast majority recover completely. However, some of the patients who seemingly recovered from acute CO poisoning may suffer delayed neurological damage. The clinical management of carbon monoxide poisoning presents a great challenge for clinicians who have to treat the acute poisoning and to reduce delayed complications.

One of the basic questions is whether to treat or not to treat carbon monoxide poisoning with HBO? It is still under discussion in the U.S.A. Only 1,500 cases are treated annually in hyperbaric chambers. In some states HBO is not used for acute CO poisoning. Doctor L.K. Weaver from LDS hospital in Salt Lake City states that at least 10,000 new cases of cognitive sequelae occur per year in the United States. HBOT should reduce the number of those who develop neurological complications by 50%.

Some Typical Errors in CO Poisoning Diagnosis and Treatment

Our experience allows us to give some advice on how to manage patients with CO poisoning.

Don't forget about the possibility of CO poisoning during the summer.

The correct diagnosis is more likely made in the winter months or when a patient is a victim of fire. In the summer months CO poisoning is often disregarded and the clinical findings are attributed to other reasons. Gastrointestinal and flu-like symptoms are often "guilty" of delaying a CO poisoning diagnosis and correct treatment.

Skin color

Some physicians look for cherry-red coloration of the skin and mucous membranes as a typical clinical sign. It is a very rare finding and should not be expected. We have seen it in some very young children and rarely in adults.

Delay in applying HBO treatment

Some argue that HBO should be applied only during the first 6 hours after rescue from the CO environment, because after this interval it would not be effective. We accept all symptomatic patients for HBO treatment, regardless the delay between the rescue of the patient from the scene and his arrival at the hyperbaric center. We have seen symptoms improve even after more than 12 hours! So, HBO is effective after 12 hours and more. We advise that all patients that reach a hyperbaric facility be treated.

How to evaluate carboxyhemoglobin levels

High levels of carboxyhemoglobin prove a severe poisoning. However, low levels do not mean that the patient is out of danger, they merely evidence that the patient was exposed to carbon monoxide. Two months ago an emergency physician asked us to prepare the chamber for a patient with 58% of carboxyhemoglobin, an almost certainly fatal level. While a patient waited for the transfer, he received oxygen by mask. Three hours later his COHb lowered till 16%, so the doctor decided not to send him to the hyperbaric chamber. It was a mistake, because this patient had a very high risk to develop neurologic complications.

Pay attention to elderly patients

While 72% of our patients are children and young adults up to 30 years of age, people over 60 compose only 4.5% of the treated group. So, in the older age group this condition is under-diagnosed. In the same family, the children are admitted to the hospital, whereas the grandparents not. Elderly patients need special attention at the time of primary care if they complain of headache, fatigue or dizziness, or if they show symptoms like unsteady gait.

Conclusions

- Hyperbaric oxygen is very efficient in the management of acute and chronic carbon monoxide poisoning victims. Patients with severe poisoning, with a history of loss of consciousness should receive this treatment. Only in patients without any symptoms, the carboxyhemoglobin level should be used as indication for HBO treatment.

- Treatment with pure oxygen in hyperbaric chamber helps to prevent neurological sequelae in carbon monoxide poisoned patients.
- If a delayed neurologic syndrome after CO poisoning is present, the patient needs treatment with hyperbaric oxygen.

Radiation Necrosis

Radiotherapy is used as part of cancer treatment combined with surgery, chemotherapy, and hormone therapy. Sometimes it is applied to reduce a cancer before surgery, or to prevent the recurrence of malignancy after its surgical elimination. For some cancer types, when its surgical removal is not possible, it is the only method of treatment.

Malignant cells or tumor cells are capable of growing more rapidly than normal cells. This enables them to invade other tissues and organs, spreading through lymphatic fluid and/or blood, and depositing in other areas of the body forming metastasis. Radiation is particularly harmful to fast-growing cells so it is more destructive for tumor cells. Unfortunately, normal cells with rapid reproduction can also die because of this process. This is the case with skin and hair that suffer so obviously from the radiation. A few weeks after the start of radiotherapy the skin is turning red, then desquamation of external layers, swelling, ulcerations, pain, and bleeding might occur. Radiation burn can also be observed. And since hair follicles

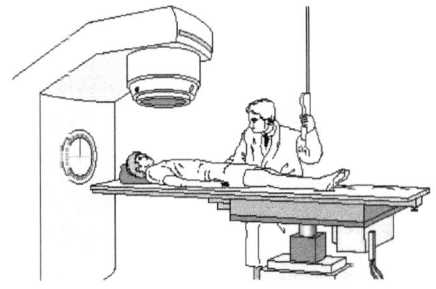

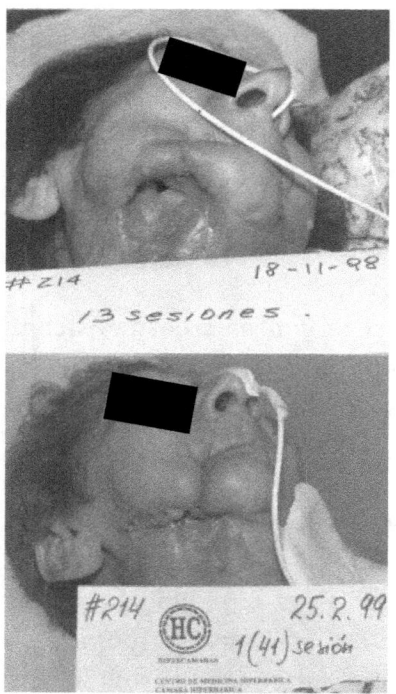

Patient with radiation ulcer before and after treatment in a hyperbaric chamber.

are very sensitive to radiation treatment hair loss may ensue.

Some time after radiation these side effects decrease or disappear. However, months or years after radiation a late complication may emerge. Radiation necrosis, a death of healthy tissue occurs, usually at the site of the original tumor. Why?

The reason is that radiotherapy affects normal cells. The most sensitive to radiation among non-tumor cells are cells which produce tissue structural framework, and cells that line the interior surface of blood vessels. Disabled by radiotherapy, these cells stop functioning normally and are unable to reproduce. As fewer cells remain in the irradiated area, organs weaken and tissues become hypocellular. Failing capillaries lead to oxygen deficiency, known as hypoxia.

This phenomenon is called "three-H": hypocellular, hypovascular, and hypoxic tissues. The result is a residual tissue with a capillary density of only 20 to 40% of normal non-radiated organs. Additionally, the tissue now consists of cells that do not reproduce themselves but die without replacement. This condition is called radionecrosis.

The influx of oxygen to these tissues during treatment in a hyperbaric chamber facilitates capillary growth and cell recovery. This effect, described first by Dr. Robert Marx from the University of Miami School of Medicine, is unique in therapeutics. The tissues are receiving more oxygen, which enhances cell recovery and the formation of the new capillaries called "neoangiogenesis", and healing. There is no other treatment that makes it possible to restore normal blood circulation in irradiated tissue.

> En la radionecrosis, el oxígeno hiperbárico es la mejor terapia posible.

This treatment has received worldwide acceptance by the medical community and is listed by the Undersea and Hyperbaric Medicine Society (UHMS)—the international leader for studies in this field of medicine—as approved for reimbursement. For example, Medicare covers HBO therapy for 15 conditions, among them soft tissue radionecrosis and osteoradionecrosis. This is possible because evidence based medicine reports facts that justify this treatment. There are more than 100 scientific papers (more than 75 in English) that describe favorable outcomes of HBO application in radiation necrosis treatment.

The Effect of Hyperbaric Oxygen on Radiated Tissue

During the first 6-8 hyperbaric sessions, no change is seen. However, using the microscope one can observe capillary budding. This is the primary mechanism of the repair process. Endothelial cells of remaining vessels begin to divide forming new capillaries. Blood begins to flow through them, bringing oxygen and nutrients necessary to form new cells capable of producing collagen. After 10-12 sessions this process accelerates, and after 20-24 sessions the proliferation continues until 75 to 85% of former capillaries reappear in the radiated zone. For years after hyperbaric oxygen treatment, these capillaries are maintained making the previously radiated tissue viable.

Radionecrosis of the Jaw

Jaw cancer belongs to the oral or mouth cancer group, which is the largest group in the head and neck cancer category. While some think this is a rare cancer, is it not so rare. Approximately 36,000 new cases of oral cancer were newly diagnosed in the population of the US in 2010. That means 100 new individuals each day. Every hour of every day one person dies from oral cancer in the US. When found at early stages of development, mouth cancers can be cured in 80 to 90% of patients.

However, 3-10% of cured patients will later develop radionecrosis of soft tissues or of bone, called osteoradionecrosis (ORN), or bone death. The above mentioned Dr. Marx created a protocol for the treatment of radionecrosis, consisting of surgery and the use of the hyperbaric oxygen therapy.

From research data and his clinical experience, he proposed as the most effective treatment the application of 20 sessions of HBO at 2.4 ATA 90 minutes each before surgery and 10 more after surgery. Bone defects require longer treatment to restore the capillary flow and cell recovery, therefore 30 HBO applications are needed before surgery and 10 following it. The soft tissue protocol is called 20/10 and the osteoradionecrosis (ORN) protocol 30/10.

"The hyperbaric oxygen therapy has revolutionized facial bone reconstruction of radiated patients because it made outcomes predictable and functional"—Dr. Marx said.

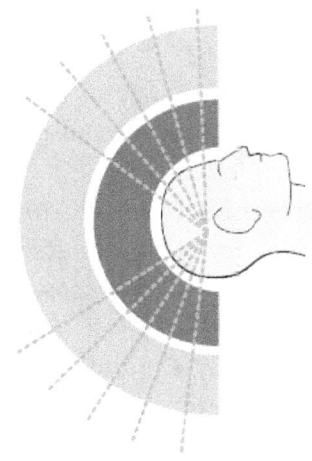

Prevention of Osteoradionecrosis of the Jaw

Osteoradionecrosis, or bone death, is perhaps the most severe radiation therapy side effect. It develops because radiation diminishes the bone's ability to withstand trauma and to avoid infection. With time, the radiated bone becomes more and more fragile. The most common cause of trauma is the removal of teeth. In the 89% of patients with trauma-induced ORN, teeth extraction was the cause of it.

Dr. Marx recommends the application of 20 HBO sessions before and 10 after teeth extraction in patients with history of jaw irradiation. This procedure improves bone capillary density and cell metabolism, therefore preventing osteoradionecrosis.

Laryngeal Radionecrosis

About 12,000 new cases of throat cancers (particularly laryngeal cancer) occur per year in the US population. Nobody is exempt from this disease. News reports show that even the famous American actor Michael Douglas is fighting throat cancer.

Treatment depends on the stage and the precise location of the cancer. For early-stage tumors, doctors may use either surgery or radiation therapy. For advanced laryngeal cancer radiation therapy is commonly combined with chemotherapy as the primary treatment. These treatments almost always have significant side effects. Surgery often affects swallowing and speaking while radiotherapy produces necrosis in some patients.

Necrosis of the larynx, also called the voice box, is a very tough radiotherapy complication. Medical treatment offers only symptomatic and temporary relief, which requires additional surgery. The nonviable tissue should be removed to promote healing. As the vocal cords are located within these tissues, patients inevitably loose their voice after the removal of the larynx.

Laryngectomy can be avoided by the application of hyperbaric oxygen. London and colleagues from the University of Virginia Medical Center in Charlottesville, US, managed to save the larynx in five patients with larynx cartilage necrosis by HBO treatment. Ferguson, Feldmeier and Filntisis, from separate institutions achieved similar outcomes. The combined results of their studies assign 34 saved larynxes in 40 patients. Most of them preserved good voice quality.

One year ago José, a man in his sixties, very thin and depressed, entered my examining room for first time. Fifteen years ago he had cancer of the vocal cords and received radiotherapy. The cancer was cured, but in three years he suffered the same type of tumor in his cheek, verified by histological study (microscopic study that permits cancer identification). Four years later he got cancer in the jaw. He survived such a complex case: two recurrences of tumor treated by radiotherapy. Now he has another problem: radionecrosis of the larynx. He lives with a tracheostomy—an opening in the trachea with an inserted tube to facilitate passage of air to the lungs. This tube was necessary because the tissues of José's trachea were swollen and devitalized. His voice was almost imperceptible. The skin around the neck opening was reddish and irritated, and the affected zone produced purulent secretions.

He was offered a surgical solution—removal of the larynx—but José refused it. Then we decided to apply hyperbaric oxygen therapy. After the 30th session he began to improve his general state, gained weight, and the purulent secretion disappeared. The healing process had begun. Although he is not completely cured, his physician notes an improvement. José has returned to his work, he is full of energy nowadays, and even though his voice is harsh he is no longer speechless.

Virginia had no luck with her laryngeal necrosis. Although she received 30 HBO applications, there was no clinical success. A recurrence of tumor was suspected, so a biopsy was done taking a small part of the affected tissue and examining it under the microscope. The return of the tumor was confirmed.

Here is an important issue to mention: biopsy acts as a micro trauma that can by itself induce necrosis, so it is undertaken only when a reappearance of tumor is suspected. The correct medical plan of treatment is: first hyperbaric oxygen, and if it is not effective, a biopsy.

Head and Neck Necrosis

The previously mentioned Dr. Marx treated 160 patients with head and neck necrosis by means of soft tissue flaps to reconstruct remnant defects. Half of them underwent

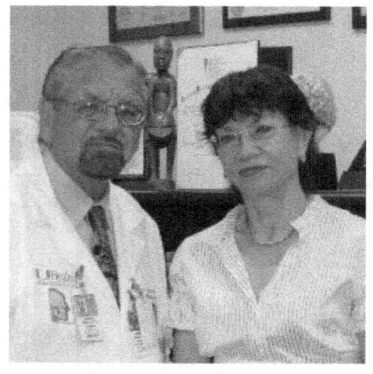
Doctor Robert Marx from the University of Miami and the author.

only surgery, while others 80 patients also received HBO 20/10 protocol. The analysis of the outcome included three wound complications aspects: wound dehiscence, which means separation of the layers of a surgical wound, wound infection and delayed healing.

The results were different in the HBO treated group versus non-treated group:

	HBO Treated	Not Treated
Wound infection	6%	24%
Wound dehiscence	11%	48%
Delayed healing	11%	55%

Delayed healing was a result of infection or of wound dehiscence. Dr. Marx wrote that the result was striking: five times more complications in the control group that didn't receive hyperbaric oxygen therapy.

Chest Wall Necrosis

Chest wall radiation necrosis occurs in breast, lung or esophageal cancers. In young women, a less radical breast cancer surgery is performed, which permits saving the breast. After this kind of surgery radiotherapy is inevitable. Carl and his colleagues from the University of Düsseldorf, Germany, published in 2001 the outcome in 44 patients with chest wall necrosis after breast-conserving surgery and radiotherapy for early breast cancer.

Thirty-two patients underwent hyperbaric oxygen treatment. Twelve formed a control group because they rejected receiving HBOT. The treated group reported pain reduction, decreasing of edema, and decrease of erythema or redness of the skin caused by blood congestion. Seven women experienced complete recovery from symptoms while patients in the control group stayed symptomatic throughout the study.

The outcome for patients with this condition is better when HBO is applied

Radiation Cystitis

Late radiation cystitis can appear from 6 months to 20 years after radiation therapy. Patients suffer from hematuria, or blood in urine, which may vary from mild to severe hemorrhage, urinary incontinence, fistula formation and bladder necrosis. If the hemorrhagic cystitis does not respond to conservative measures, it may require bladder removal. There are many reports of positive outcomes in 60 to 95% of patients treated with HBO.

Horacio, 68, received radiotherapy for prostate cancer. Eight years later symptoms of radiation cystitis presented. He suffered pain during urination, frequent urination and desire to urinate without results. The situation was getting worse and hematuria emerged. It was a hemorrhagic cystitis in a severe form—Horacio practically urinated blood. He received repeated blood transfusions, which in a few hours turned up in his urine bag.

The reason was a typical lesion induced by previous radiation. The inner layer of the bladder is very sensitive to radiation and became hypocellular, hypovascular, hypoxic. This inner lining of the bladder practically disappeared, denuding the capillaries or tiny blood vessels. So all the inner surface of the bladder was bleeding due to shallow superficial multiple lesions. What is the best treatment? Hyperbaric oxygen. After 15 HBO applications the hemorrhage began to diminish. After 30 sessions the bladder stopped bleeding.

Amelia received radiotherapy because of uterine cervix tumor or tumor of the lower, narrow portion of the uterus (womb) where it joins with the top end of the vagina. She also suffered massive hemorrhages and also got better with hyperbaric oxygen treatment. When she seemed to be cured the hemorrhage recurred. This time she was losing pure red blood of arterial origin. Almost all the bladder surface was cured, but one artery of medium size was shedding blood. An interventional radiologist delivered small particles of a synthetic material called an embolic agent through a special catheter to this artery, which stopped the bleeding.

Amelia's case reveals the importance of multidisciplinary approach in medicine. To stop bleeding from the capillaries the HBO application was needed, while massive hemorrhage from one artery required a procedure called embolization.

Radiation Enteritis and Proctitis

Chronic proctitis and enteritis are complications of pelvic irradiation. Often months or years later, radiotherapy damages the lining of the intestines (bowels). The patient suffers from diarrhea, bleeding or mucus from the rectum, feeling the need to have a bowel movement most or all of the time, pain in the rectal area, especially during bowel movements. Other symptoms can include: loss of appetite, nausea and vomiting, stomach cramping or pain. The late symptoms include stricture, fistulae, perforations, ulcerations of the bowel wall and gross hemorrhages.

So the lining of the intestines should be treated. There are few options for this: or surgical removal of part of affected intestine, or superficial desiccation or coagulation of the lining with endoscopic laser, electrical current or formalin. All these methods eliminate the damaged tissue. Hyperbaric oxygen tries to restore it.

Doctor J.J. Feldmeier from medical College of Ohio, Toledo, Ohio, a well-known specialist in oncology and hyperbaric medicine, in 2004 reviewed 114 such cases treated with HBO, among them 41 (36%) cases cured and 68 (60%) improved, in six out of eight cases fistulae were resolved as well.

The outcome in patients who received HBO therapy is better than after any other treatment.

Neurologic Radiation Injuries

More than 40,000 new cases of brain tumors are diagnosed in US each year. They are treated with stereotactic radiosurgery or with radiotherapy. The first is a one-session non-invasive treatment performed with a Gamma Knife instrument. During treatment many beams of radiation enter the brain, precisely targeted to the tumor location point. In cases where radiosurgery is unacceptable, radiotherapy is used. It consists of many radiation sessions. Another medical indication for application of radiation is cerebral arteriovenous malformation (AVM). AVM is an abnormal connection between arteries and veins in the brain, most commonly formed before birth. Normally, blood passes from arteries through capillaries to be collected in veins. In an AVM blood goes directly from arteries to veins through the abnormal vessels that could have very thin walls with high risk of sudden bleeding because of their fragility. AVMs are detected in more than 25,000 Americans per year. Stereotactic radiosurgery has been widely used on small AVMs with considerable success. But 8 to10% of patients develop long term neurological symptoms after radiation, many of them radionecrosis of the brain.

The standard treatment of cerebral radionecrosis includes surgical exploration for removal of the necrotic part and medical therapy with corticosteroids, both with limited success. The analysis made in 2004 by Dr. Feldmeier of 63 clinical cases reported by different authors, showed a positive outcome confirmed by neuroimaging studies in 29 patients (46%) treated with HBO application. And in 27 of 29 patients it was possible to reduce the amount of steroids requirement. In 2009, physicians in Spain reported three successful cases of brain radionecrosis treated with hyperbaric oxygen. Wanebo JE, from San Diego, US, described other six favorable cases in the same year.

It is worth mentioning that hyperbaric oxygen treatment should be initiated early. The clinical cases of HBO application in radiation induced optical neuritis reported by Guy and Schatz from University of Florida in Gainesville, USA, show better outcomes in visual function when hyperbaric oxygen treatment was begun within 72 hours of vision loss. Patients who began HBO 2 to 6 weeks after vision loss had no improvement.

Our patient Maria had brain hemorrhage because of AVM rupture and was treated by radiosurgery in two areas, according to the location of malformations. Everything seemed to be excellent, but Maria entered the small group of patients that develop radionecrosis around the area of the surgery. One year after the intervention she began to lose sight in half of the field of vision, first in one eye and then in another. This condition is called homonymous hemianopsia. It was not an eye defect, but a brain failure, the brain being responsible for recognizing visual images. Two months passed from the first symptoms to the beginning of HBO sessions. This was probably the reason for not achieving any clinical success in this case.

While Maria received HBO treatment, she developed another radionecrosis in the motor cortex, where the second surgery had taken place. Suddenly she could not move one leg, it became paralyzed, and Maria fell to the floor. A brain MRI showed another necrotic zone. After 40 HBO sessions Maria practically recovered voluntary movement in her leg. It seems that this time the successful outcome was due to the immediate start of treatment.

We observed a positive outcome in another patient treated for the same reason. We recorded him walking before and after 30 HBO sessions, documenting the success of the treatment on video tape.

It seems that the beneficial effect of hyperbaric oxygen in treatment of radiation induced brain necrosis is due not only to oxygenation, but also to some others mechanisms. Doctor Steven Thom, a researcher from the University of Pennsylvania found in 2006 that HBO mobilizes stem cells from the bone marrow and enhances their availability in circulating blood. This phenomenon could probably add to the positive outcome in patients with cerebral necrosis treated by HBO.

It is very difficult to treat this group of patients because of complications that are typical in this pathology. In patients who have brain tumors, local cerebral edema or radiation necrosis, oxygen induced seizures during HBOT are more common than in any other group of patients, because of the necrotic areas in their brain that trigger episodic similar abnormal electrical activity in the neurons as found in patients with epilepsy. In some of our patients we have observed convulsions even with normobaric oxygen, before chamber pressurization.

We have had to invent a special protocol for these patients, gradually increasing the chamber pressure from one HBO session to another in order to "train" them to accept greater oxygen partial pressures. In some cases we had to add antioxidants intake, such as vitamin E. Anticonvulsant medication may also need to be increased to ensure that it's levels are sufficient to prevent seizures, a severe HBO complication.

The incidence of oxygen induced seizures in the US is very low: 1 case in 10,000 patient treatments. We have observed it even less often: 1 in 25,000 patient sessions and only in patients with cerebral necrosis.

Hyperbaric Oxygen as Radiosensitizer

From the 1950s to the 1970s, hyperbaric oxygen was used as a radiosensitizer. This word means to enhance the sensitivity of tumor tissues to radiotherapy. Being hypoxic, the majority of tumor tissues are resistant to radiation therapy. The British physician and researcher, Dr. Churchill-Davidson, first had the idea of combining HBOT and radiotherapy. Oxygen received in a hyperbaric chamber is a very potent radiosensitizer. At the same time it is the least toxic agent used for sensitization of radiotherapy.

For technical reasons and lacking a protocol to achieve comparable results, this method was abandoned. However, in recent years Japanese physicians have begun to use hyperbaric oxygenation before radiotherapy. Radiotherapy given within 15 minutes after an HBO treatment is more efficient because the body still retains 100% oxygen before it is gradually replaced by ambient air.

> HBO doesn't generate malignant growth. Patients with cancer that need HBO should not be deprived of this treatment.

In Europe, at Amsterdam University's Children Cancer Center there is a favorable experience of neuroblastoma treatment with HBO inclusion in the therapeutic scheme.

Hyperbaric Oxygen Doesn't Promote Tumor Growth

For many years, physicians wondered if hyperbaric oxygen – while enhancing cell growth – would also increase cancer cell development. Patients with radionecrosis are at high risk for recurring cancer, either because of formation of a new tumor or incomplete eradication of the existing one.

In many cases, the same reason that provoked cancer persists. The example of smoking patients is very demonstrative. According to statistics, 83% of smokers do not quit smoking after cancer treatment and 33% of smokers cured of cancer develop another tumor within five years.

In 2001, a Lisbon consensus conference supported by the European Society of Radiation Therapy and Oncology

(ESTRO) and by the European Committee of Hyperbaric Medicine (ECHM), determined the effectiveness of hyperbaric oxygen in radiation lesions. Some scientific papers have shown that hyperbaric oxygen not only does not promote cancer, but also reduces the formation of metastasis. Tumors that receive insufficient oxygen respond less to cancer treatment, have an aggressive growth, and produce more lethal metastasis.

There is scientific evidence that HBO would not generate malignant growth. So, patients with cancer who need HBO should not be deprived of this treatment. We can actually say that hyperbaric oxygen provides a protective effect against tumors. It is worth remembering the words of a famous Russian physician, Dr. Pahkomov: "We should bathe tumor with oxygen".

Present and Future of HBOT in Late Radiation Pathology

Hyperbaric oxygen is recommended as an adjunct treatment for radiation injuries of many organs. The aim of HBO treatment is to recover damaged tissues. The alternative is surgery or others method to eliminate compromised tissue, which in many cases reduces the quality of life.

Baromedical Research Foundation in Columbia, South Carolina, USA, is a leader in a multicenter randomized controlled clinical study known as HORTIS (Hyperbaric Oxygen Radiation Tissue Injury Study). When it is finished, physicians will have evidence based proof of how and when to use the HBO in radiation damage of the jaw, larynx, skin, bladder, rectum, bowel and gynecological area

The Cochrane Collaboration, a nongovernmental institution provides reviews of scientific advances. In its last issue it recognizes HBO treatment for post radiation lesions of head, neck, anus and rectum.

ASEPTIC BONE NECROSIS

Carina is a girl aged 23 who has been suffering from right hip pain for a year. She has been on crutches and taking anti-inflammatory drugs for months. Little by little she is getting worse. The reason? Aseptic necrosis of the femoral head. The femur is the long bone that carries the weight of our body and enables us to walk.

The traumatologist proposed surgery with an uncertain outcome. Then, Carina found us in the Internet. Her medical insurance company didn't cover the HBO treatment for this pathology, but Carina didn't give up and asked for the protection of her rights before a judge, who ordered the insurance company to pay for the treatment. We began to treat her. At first, the pain subsided and later disappeared completely. After 38 HBO applications Carina was healed. A forensic medical expert evaluated the images of her femoral head and assessed a complete recovery. How

> The best treatment from the initial stages of avascular bone necrosis is hyperbaric oxygen therapy. Oxygen is necessary for viability, as well as bone repair and remodeling.

many other patients may require the same treatment?

In the United States, approximately 15,000 new cases of avascular bone necrosis are reported each year, mostly in people between 30 and 60 years of age. Almost 90% of these patients suffer it in the hip joint. Avascular necrosis, called also aseptic necrosis, osteonecrosis or ischemic bone necrosis, involves cellular death of bone components. It occurs when there is an interruption of circulation to some parts of the bone. It affects bones with a single terminal blood supply, such as the femoral head, femoral condyles and humerus. These bones have limited collateral circulation. So knee and shoulder joints are also among the mostly affected. If the patient is not treated, the bone collapses, and the joint deteriorates. The process is almost always progressive, leading to joint destruction within five years.

Avascular bone necrosis sometimes is due to an underlying disease or direct trauma, such as a fracture that affects blood supply to the bone. It can also develop after corticosteroids administration, excessive alcohol consumption, radiation therapy, or decompression illness. Other diseases that may result in avascular necrosis include diabetes, atherosclerosis and gout. In many cases it is not associated with trauma or disease, so it is called "idiopathic", that means arising spontaneously or from an unknown cause. This was the case with Carina.

A similar condition is the disease of Legg-Calvé-Perthes, also named coxa plana or Legg-Perthes disease (LCPD, or Perthes). It is found only in children between the ages of 2 and 12, most frequently boys. It is a form of osteonecrosis of the hip or of the femoral head. There are many theories, but in fact the origin of LCPD is still unknown.

Symptoms of Avascular Necrosis of the Femoral Head

Unfortunately, avascular necrosis may initially be asymptomatic and is occasionally discovered incidentally on radiographs. With bone damage progression, pain appears in the affected joint. Pain increases progressively worsening over time and joint use. When the bone collapses, joint movement is restricted and the patient begins to limp.

Treatment

Treatment depends on the underlying cause. Patients are medicated with anti-inflammatory non-steroidal drugs. To limit weight bearing, crutches are prescribed. In most cases surgery is needed, ranging from bone grafting to total joint replacement. Despite advances in orthopedic surgery, most patients with advanced avascular bone necrosis require more than one total hip replacement during their lifetime.

The best treatment in the initial stages of avascular bone necrosis is hyperbaric oxygen therapy. Oxygen is necessary for viability, healing and bone regeneration. The beneficial effects of oxygen on bone formation, mobilization of bone precursors, and fracture healing are well documented. During HBOT, dying bone cells receive high concentration oxygen through plasma instead of erythrocytes.

This therapy, consisting of about 60-100 HBO treatments at 2.2-2.5 ATA, saves affected tissues, helps to reabsorb non-viable tissues, and heals bone defects.

Clinical Outcomes of Avascular Bone Necrosis Treatment in Adults

Dr. Michael Strauss at Long Beach Memorial Medical Center in California, USA, studied 4,224 cases of avascular bone necrosis appearing in medical journals. He selected only papers containing imaging confirmation of therapeutic results. He classified the outcome as successful when joint mobility was restored and pain reduced. In 3,193 cases treated with surgery, there were successful outcomes in 66% of the cases. In 189 cases treated with the inclusion of hyperbaric oxygen therapy, excellent results were observed in 81%. Treatment modalities might complement one another. For example, cephalic decompression surgery diminishes internal pressure in the bone while HBO stimulates the growth of new blood vessels promoting bone regeneration. Both techniques contribute to the healing process.

Clinical Outcomes of Legg-Calvé-Perthes Disease Treatment

Cuban physicians applied HBO to 210 patients with Perthes disease. The patients received three series of 15, 10 and 10 HBO treatments separated with 7 weeks between each. Some patients required an additional series of 10 treatments. Generally, the healing time for this condition is three years. In this study 92% of patients were cured in less than two years.

Treatment cost

In 1997, Dr. Strauss showed the benefits of HBO in avascular bone necrosis focusing on the cost-benefit relationship. While the high number of HBO sessions required may be costly, other options are even more expensive. For example, a hip prosthesis may need to be replaced surgically every 5-10 years. The younger the patient, the greater the total cost.

Sudden Deafness and Acoustic Trauma

Spontaneous hearing impairment without any apparent cause, which occurs suddenly or over a period of up to three days, is called sudden deafness or sensorineural hearing loss. It might affect anybody: from children and young adults (20-30 years) to middle-aged and older persons. Approximately 4, 000 new cases of sudden hearing loss occur annually in the United States, and 15,000 are reported in other counties. According to German data, each year there are 20 new cases per 100,000 people. The number of new cases during some time period is called incidence. Japanese researchers noted that incidence of sudden deafness increases with age: in people over fifty is three-fold that in young adults. No differences were found between sexes.

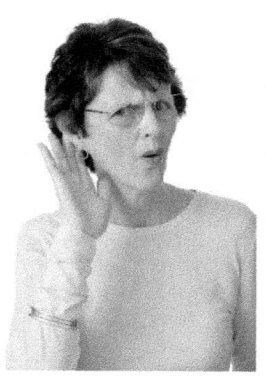

The deafness appears suddenly: patients in good general health relate that they noticed it when they woke up in the morning or picked up the phone trying to use the damaged ear. Or they report hear ringing of different intensity in the absence of acoustic stimuli, something like "white noise" in that ear. It appears to be stronger at night when ambient noise decreases. This false perception of sound is called tinnitus. Other symptoms are dizziness, vertigo, and nausea. Some patients can perceive a short quick explosive "pop" before hearing loss.

What Causes Sudden Hearing Loss?

> Hyperbaric oxygen therapy is useful for the treatment of sudden deafness and tinnitus, as long as the patient is treated in the first two weeks, and is also acceptable within the first three months after onset.

There are many possible causes of sudden deafness, but in each clinical case it is very difficult to identify precisely the specific cause. It could be due to an inflammation of the inner ear, a viral infection, a vasospasm or constriction of blood vessels of the inner ear. It may also be due to vascular occlusion caused by a blood clot (thrombus) or by a small piece of fat tissue. Other causes can be: hemorrhage, allergic disorders, metabolic problems, stress, and injury of the anatomical structures of the ear. All these conditions inhibit the blood flow to auditory sensory cells, which are responsible for sound perception in the inner ear, so there is lack of oxygen needed for normal acoustic function.

It is assumed that the immune system is involved in this pathology, because in the blood of about half of these patients different pathological antibodies were found. In addition, some patients with sudden deafness suffer from fatigue, muscle pain, joint pain, depression, diarrhea, fibromyalgia and chronic fatigue syndrome. Sometimes they attribute the loss of hearing to respiratory congestion from a cold or to allergy.

Clinical cases that occur without apparent cause doctors call "idiopathic". Idiopathic means arising spontaneously or from an unknown cause. Most sudden deafness cases are idiopathic.

Anyhow it is assumed that there is inflammation, swelling (edema), decreased circulation and lack of oxygen or hypoxia.

Spontaneous Recovery

The prognosis in cases of sudden sensorineural hearing loss is generally good, and the spontaneous improvement within a matter of days is common. Some patients recover without medical treatment within the first three days. Others can get better during the first or second week. But patients in whom there is no change within two weeks are unlikely to show much recovery. With time they are getting worse.

Why to Treat Sudden Deafness in a Hyperbaric Chamber?

Traditional treatment includes drugs that reduce inflammation and improve circulation by opening the arteries and preventing inappropriate blood clotting. Therefore, therapy includes steroids, vasodilators, plasma expanders, anticoagulants and antivirals.

A hyperbaric chamber delivers more oxygen to tissues, enhancing energy production in cells and at the same time

> Treatment of acute acoustic trauma with hyperbaric chamber and steroids is effective only if hyperbaric oxygen therapy is started within ten days of the accident.

helping to combat infections because of the "antibiotic" properties of pure oxygen.

In addition, hyperbaric oxygen (HBO) improves the state of the immune system, promotes healing by various very important effects: it down regulates different substances that are involved in inflammation and acts as intracellular signal transducer and modulator of cellular gene functions. The cells that were almost dead from hypoxia, or lack of oxygen, begin to awake and produce growth factors, antioxidant enzymes and many others protective substances.

Statistics about Treatment

Otolaryngologists from the University of Pisa, Italy, assigned 30 patients with sudden sensorineural deafness referred to their clinic within the first 48 hours of symptom onset, to once-daily administration of hyperbaric oxygen for ten days. Another 20 patients were treated during ten days with only intravenous vasodilators, or medications that open the arteries and thereby increase blood flow. After completion of therapy patients treated in a hyperbaric chamber showed greater improvement than those who received vasodilators.

According to another study conducted in Turkey, and published in 2004 in the European Archives of Otorhinolaryngology, the group of patients treated with hyperbaric oxygen therapy plus medication had a greater hearing gain than those not treated in the chamber and receiving only medication. The beneficial effect was more pronounced in patients younger than 50 years.

German doctors in 1998 reviewed the results of treatment in more than 4000 patients with sudden deafness of unknown cause or acoustic trauma. They confirmed that

65% of those patients treated in a combined approach with hyperbaric oxygen and conventional pharmacologic therapy demonstrated a hearing improvement.

Furthermore, studies in Japan, Germany, Croatia, Russia and other countries showed that hyperbaric oxygen therapy is useful if applied early, ideally within the first two weeks, and acceptable within the first three months. Once six months have passed, treatment is ineffective.

We always regret when we receive young patients referred late for hyperbaric treatment. We do not reject them because statistics and our experience show that some of them may still benefit.

Some doctors suggest starting treatment with steroids, and, if the patient does not respond, only then apply HBOT. This treatment model is acceptable if steroids are shown to be ineffective and the patient is referred to the hyperbaric chamber during the first two weeks from the time he or she became aware of diminished hearing.

Acoustic Trauma

Acoustic trauma is hearing loss caused by loud noise (nearby explosion, gunfire, machinery noise, etc.). Acoustic trauma affects blood circulation in the inner ear. The hyperbaric chamber provides more oxygen to the tissues, so its timely use can reduce hearing loss or heal it.

According to Pilgramm and Schumann, German otolaryngologists, hyperbaric oxygen therapy in this condition is more successful than any other treatment modality.

Dr. Okamoto and his colleagues in Japan demonstrated in 2005 that the treatment of acute acoustic trauma with steroids and hyperbaric oxygen is effective only if hyperbaric oxygen therapy is started within the first 10 days after the accident.

Our Experience

We treated over 100 patients with sudden deafness and tinnitus (a few presented acoustic trauma) in a period of twelve years. Fifty percent of them were males. Besides hearing loss 50% of the patients suffered tinnitus; some had vertigo, dizziness, nausea, vomiting and other vestibular signs.

> In 2005, the organization Cochrane Collaboration found evidence that hearing can be improved and that tinnitus can be reduced if hyperbaric oxygen treatment is applied during the first two weeks of onset of symptoms.

Interval between onset of symptoms and beginning of HBO varied from three days to more than one year. According to bibliographic data, the majority of our patients had no chance for spontaneous improvement.

The age of our patients varied from 13 to 79 years, the largest group being 50-59 years of age, exactly as worldwide statistics indicate. Our patients received standard therapy, which included steroids and vasodilators. HBO was given once a day at 2.0 ATA for 60 minutes.

Twenty patients didn't complete five sessions; they were eliminated from the analyses. They chose to discontinue HBO treatment, and in our experience, patients with this pathology are more prone to reject chamber treatment than others. Most likely they feared difficulty equalizing the pressure in their already compromised ears. But statistics show that ear complications occur more frequently in patients with head and neck radionecrosis than in this group.

Eighty-two patients completed more than five sessions. Sixty-eight percent of them reported subjective improvement with combined therapy that was objectively confirmed by audiometry in 45%. Tinnitus was also reduced. The improvement varied from 15 dB in some patients to complete recovery in two cases.

Fifty-five percent of patients didn't recover their auditory function. Among them some improved tinnitus.

> A reliable diagnosis is achieved with an audiometric study. The hearing loss is measured in decibels (dB) at different frequencies of sound. The decibel scale measures how loud a sound is with 60 dB corresponding to the loudness of normal conversation. Frequency is another sound characteristic measured as high or low in the scale. Frequency is measured in number of cycles per second or hertz (Hz). In normal conversation the frequency of sound varies from 500 to 3000 Hz. The U.S. National Institute on Deafness and Other Communication Disorders, defines sudden deafness as hearing loss of 30 dB or more (measured in 3 audiometric frequencies) if this loss appears within 72 hours in individuals without previous hearing problems. If it comes at a time longer than 72 hours it is called "rapidly progressive hearing loss."

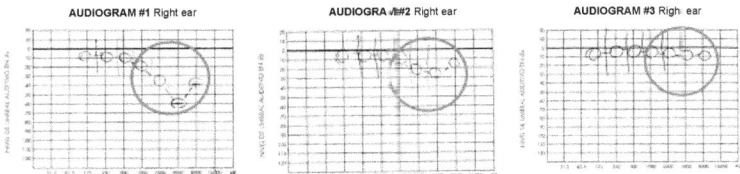

The audiogram shows the level of sound required to be just audible.
First audiogram: hearing loss 60 dB, before HBOT.
Second audiogram: partial recovery of hearing after 1 week of HBOT (30 dB)
Third testing: recovery of hearing after 2 weeks of HBOT.

Why some patients did not show any improvement? The factor reported in bibliography as most important is the interval between the appearance of symptoms and the beginning of HBO treatment. The longer this interval, the less the chance for a positive outcome. So, the key to success is early HBO application.

Some physicians believe once three months have passed since the onset of deafness, patients will not respond to hyperbaric therapy. Our experience shows the possibility of hearing gain after six months of delay, but only as a partial improvement and in a lesser part of patients.

As some patients treated with delay have responded to treatment, we treat all patients sent to our Hyperbaric Center, no matter the interval since the onset of deafness. But it is much better to treat these patients as soon as possible to get a good clinical outcome.

Sudden deafness is an urgent medical problem that can range in severity from mild to profound. But as many patients are not aware of this, they tend to seek medical aid late. Since there is no pain, patients rarely worry too much about it. Since they did not suffer an obvious injury, they wait for the hearing to clear up on its own. But the delay in diagnosis and treatment may result in permanent deafness.

Conclusion

During the last 30 years hyperbaric oxygen therapy has been successfully used to treat sudden deafness, rapidly progressive hearing loss, tinnitus and acoustic trauma. In all these conditions, although of different origin, the auditory sensory cells, which are responsible for sound perception in the inner ear, have been damaged, and they may recover with hyperbaric oxygen treatment.

Recommendations

If you notice sudden decrease in hearing, consult your physician without delay. Do not wait; insist that it is an urgent medical problem that must be attended immediately. If you do not recover normal hearing in a short time with medication, ask for hyperbaric oxygen treatment.

According to statistics, almost half of patients who do not improve after the first two weeks still have a chance to restore their hearing, at least partially, if treated in a hyperbaric chamber.

Neurological Disorders

Fatigued Neurons

Human life is becoming longer. Experts from the World Health Organization estimate that in 25 years life expectancy will increase from 66 to 73 years. Will we enjoy a healthy old age?

With age there is an increase in incidence of dementia. Dementia is an impairment of brain function that affects memory, behavior, ability of learning, and communication. Slowly the signs and symptoms are getting worse. Some types of dementia are due to inadequate cerebral blood supply. In subcortical vascular dementia white matter is damaged. This dementia is called Binswanger's disease or subcortical vascular syndrome with leukoaraiosis, and it affects 1 in 4 people over 65 years of age.

Leukoaraiosis means white matter rarefaction (loss of density) seen by modern imaging techniques, such as magnetic resonance imaging (MRI). These changes are typical in persons with impaired attention, decreased working memory and inability to solve problems, slurred speech, impaired walking, balance problems, poor control of body posture, and poor control of sphincters.

The Argentine neurologist, José Vila, a specialist in this field, attributes the cause of this disease to the changes experienced by tiny blood vessels supplying blood to the brain, the capillaries, whose walls gradually lose elasticity and selective permeability. A part of the fluid transported by the capillary leaks into brain tissue and accumulates there. As a result, the distance between the capillaries and the cerebral cells increases and reduces the blood supply to the tissues. Some areas of the brain then show a lack of oxygen. This hypoxia leads to less energy production in the cells, which appear to be dormant, but actually still alive for some time. These cells can be revived by sending them hyperbaric oxygen.

In this condition, the distance the oxygen has to travel from blood vessels through brain tissue to reach the neurons, is higher than normal. The hyperbaric chamber increases the partial pressure of oxygen in blood making oxygen easily reach the most remote brain cells. Those areas are still getting little blood, but now this blood is ten-fold richer in oxygen.

We have treated many patients with this type of dementia. Our experience is that all improve, although the recovery is greater in the case of patients who had symptoms for less than a year. On average, this improvement lasts 6 to 8 months, after which it is advisable to repeat the therapy because the degenerative process continues, although at a slower pace.

Stroke

Don Julio was brought to Buenos Aires in air ambulance from a distant province. The neurologist sent him to the hyperbaric chamber because of a stroke, or cerebrovascular accident, which is a loss of brain functions due to local lack of oxygen. Don Julio was paralyzed on one side of the body and had slurred speech. He entered our Center lying on a stretcher, but progressively improved with each HBO session, and left our clinic ten days later walking without a limp and with no other neurological damage.

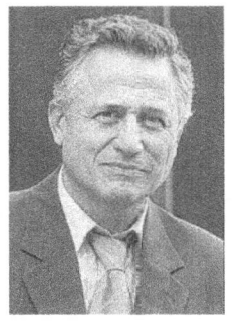

Dr. José F. Vila, a neurologist and specialist in hyperbaric medicine.

The cerebrovascular accident (CVA) is a disease caused by lack of oxygen in an area of the brain due to problems in the arteries that carry blood to the brain. The most common reason of it is atherosclerosis or "hardening of the arteries" that increases in severity with age. The stroke could be ischemic (interruption of blood flow) or hemorrhagic (leakage of blood). Don Julio had an ischemic stroke. When blood supply decreases below the critical level, brain tissue is unable to function and connected body functions also fail, leading to paralysis in one or both limbs on one side of the body, inability to speak and to understand speech, etc.

It is estimated that each year 700,000 Americans experience a stroke, new or recurrent. About 157,000 people die from strokes each year, the third leading cause of death after heart disease and cancer.

To understand the effects of HBO in stroke or cerebral infarct, we need to explain the processes that take place in the brain during stroke. The acute loss of perfusion (pumping blood into a tissue) to any zone of the brain results in ischemia and neuronal death. The larger the artery occluded the greater the brain damage and the number of neurons that die. But not all this tissue is irreversibly lost. Some peripheral parts can be rescued. These parts are called the "ischemic penumbra". The concept of ischemic penumbra appeared some thirty years ago.

Umbra and penumbra are names given to a shadow created by any light source. The umbra is a complete shadow, while the penumbra is a partial shadow, when the light source is obscured, but does not disappear.

Studying nervous tissue in the cerebral infarcts, Astrup from Denmark, Siesgo from Sweden, and Symon from United Kingdom, discovered that around the infarcted tissue (with no circulation, umbra) there is a peri-infarcted zone (penumbra), where the blood flow is diminished but still present. This reduced circulation is insufficient to permit this tissue to transmit electric signal or function normally, but enough to maintain this part of the brain alive. The neurons in this zone were called "idling". They are viable, but electrically non-functional.

These neurons need oxygen. In the presence of hyperbaric oxygen the "idling" neurons are stimulated, they are converted into metabolically active cells beginning to produce energy. This is potentially recoverable tissue.

Clinically it is very important to differentiate between idling and normal neurons. One of the modern imaging techniques named SPECT (single photon emission computerized tomography) allows us to visualize the active cells because they absorb and store a tracer used in this method. A tracer is a detectable substance introduced into a biological system. The "idling" neurons are inactive; they do not absorb the tracer. On SPECT images they are seen as blue zones. After HBO stimulation these neurons become active and begin to store the tracer. That is why after HBO they are recognized by this uptake of tracer: blue zones convert into yellow and red ones. Comparing

SPECT images of the brain before and after HBO one can observe the regions of potentially recoverable brain tissue. With the help of hyperbaric oxygen therapy, the penumbral areas are converted into normally functioning tissue.

Idling neurons are capable of surviving for some period of time. The use of HBO stimulates these metabolically lethargic and functionally inactive neurons. The hyperbaric oxygen overcomes hypoxia (lack of oxygen), reduces cerebral edema, restores cell membranes and practically saves these penumbra areas.

The best results are achieved with lower pressures and shorter sessions than those required by other conditions. The controlled study published in 1995 in the *Journal Stroke* by Dr. Nighoghossian and colleagues, showed that CVA patients who were treated with hyperbaric oxygen showed better recovery than those not treated in a hyperbaric chamber. The comparison was made one year after treatment.

The actual protocol of ischemic stroke treatment includes injection of substances to dissolve blood clots occluding the artery and inhibiting blood flow, within 3 hours of stroke onset. This procedure is called thrombolysis or lysis of thrombus.

Doctor Marc Fisher, from Worcester Memorial Hospital, Worcester, MA, advocates that modern imaging techniques permit a more precise identification of the ischemic penumbra and of stroke patients more likely to respond to delayed thrombolysis beyond the current three hour limit.

This ischemic penumbra, as we know, is responding also to HBO treatment. One should find the best protocol to combine these two techniques. Hopefully, in the near

> The lack of oxygen in certain areas of the brain results in dementia. The cells are dormant, but they may be recovered by supplying them oxygen in a hyperbaric chamber.

future, imaging identification of the ischemic penumbra will guide acute stroke therapy to target those patients most likely to respond to treatment.

Cerebral Trauma and Cerebral Ischemia

Hipoxia Cerebral hypoxia is a lack of oxygen supply to the brain, even when there is adequate blood flow. Drowning, suffocation, choking, cardiac arrest, brain trauma, carbon monoxide poisoning and complications of general anesthesia can create conditions for cerebral hypoxia. Symptoms of mild cerebral hypoxia include inattentiveness, poor decision making, memory loss and reduced motor coordination. Brain cells are extremely sensitive to total deprivation of oxygen and death can occur within five minutes. The prolonged lack of oxygen can cause coma, convulsions, and brain death.

Each year thousands of children are saved from drowning, but lack of oxygen to the brain for a long time can cause permanent neurological damage. Those children will not have a normal life and some of them will need special care permanently. If they are treated on time in a hyperbaric chamber they may be greatly helped. Brain trauma caused by accidents also produces neurological disorders.

Alejandro, a driver aged 22, was shot and taken to the hospital where a team of cardiovascular surgeons attended the emergency of a tear in the right atrium. His heart had stopped beating for eight minutes. This caused a brain injury: he did not speak, did not recognize his family and his pupils were not reacting to light. Alejandro responded only to painful stimuli. The cause was eight minutes of clinical death resulting in cerebral ischemia. After two weeks he was referred to our hyperbaric center. Gradually, over 26 sessions, he began to regain his sight and temporal and spatial orientation until, in a very emotional moment, he recognized his mother. His neurological and psychic functions were completely recovered.

At the Ocean Hyperbaric Center, in the United States, led for over 30 years by the late Dr. Neubauer, hundreds of patients have been treated with traumatic brain injury with good results.

Chronic Traumatic Brain Injury

TBI is a major cause of death and disability worldwide, especially in children and young adults. Causes include falls, vehicle accidents, and violence. It is well described in the Chapter "Severe Trauma".

In addition to the damage caused at the moment of injury, brain trauma leads to secondary damage, with a variety of events taking place in the minutes and days following the injury. These processes, which include alterations in cerebral blood flow and pressure within the skull, contribute substantially to the damage from the initial injury. The main pathophysiological mechanism of the secondary injury is hypoxia or lack of oxygenation of the affected brain.

This secondary injury can cause a host of physical, cognitive, emotional, and behavioral effects, and outcomes can range from complete recovery to permanent disability or death. A significant proportion of military personnel who have served in war retain chronic traumatic brain injury, post-traumatic brain disorders or depression. Suicide rates are high among them. A delay in treatment results in shattered lives.

Hyperbaric medicine is one of the treatments for this condition that provides excellent clinical results. Oxygen's mechanism of action is now well known. It generates new blood vessels, restores dormant cells previously deprived of oxygen, builds new bone, skin, fights infections and stimulates a patient's own stem cells. It has been used to treat brain injury from decompression sickness for over 100 years.

Dr. Paul Harch from Louisiana State University reported on military veterans treated at his facility. The veterans with blast-injuries, many with multiple concussions, experienced a 15 point IQ increase over 35 days, as measured before and after the block of hyperbaric treatments. This is the difference between a construction worker and an engineer. Post concussion syndrome was reduced by 40%, four times the amount considered clinically significant. Post Traumatic Stress disorder was reduced by 30% and depression reduced by 51%, all on standardized tests used to measure these improvements. Functional brain imaging showed restoration of brain blood flow, improvement in metabolism and recovery of useful brain tissue. All results are highly statistically significant and improvements are permanent.

In many states the medical centers are replicating Dr. Harch's work, using the same protocol. Hyperbaric medical centers in Arizona, California, Colorado, Florida, Minnesota, Oklahoma and many other states are taking part in this important scientific and clinical work. This project is called "Hyperbaric Oxygen Therapy in Chronic

Traumatic Brain Injury or Post-Traumatic Stress Disorder."

One thousand patients will be recruited. Subjects will be 18-65 years old and diagnosed with mild or moderate (not severe) TBI or Post-Traumatic Stress Disorder by either the military or civilian neurologists or neuropsychologists. This diagnosis will specially include war veterans who have had a significant decrease in their neuropsychological test scores.

Conclusion

- Hyperbaric oxygen is used in different neurological diseases and conditions.
- Vascular dementia, stroke, hypoxic or anoxic encephalopathy and mild or moderate traumatic brain injury are indications for HBO treatment.
- Neurologist should be always part of the medical staff treating these patients.
- The protocol for brain injury is of low pressure (1.5 ATA) because of the extreme sensitivity of the injured brain to any intervention.

Children with Autism

Thomas is 6 years old. He doesn't speak, doesn't obey his parents' orders, and is always trying to take his clothes off. If he doesn't want to do something, he cries "aaaaaaaaaaa…" and attempts to hide.

Oliver is a brilliant young man who graduated recently from a university in the U.S. He planned to join the Army, but then he was diagnosed as autistic. It was a surprising bit of news for those who knew him. A very intelligent boy, yet interestingly he never makes eye contact or initiates conversation – he only answers questions from others.

Generally speaking, autism is an abnormal absorption with the self; marked by short attention span and inability to interact with others, resulting in communication disorders at different levels. Within autism there are as many degrees as patients. Some patients present delays in cognitive development and language, others don't meet the full set of criteria for autism. Because of this variability, the World Health Organization classifies abnormalities in social

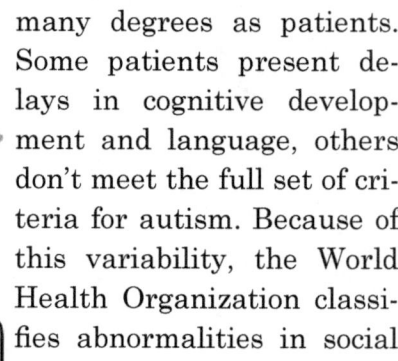

interaction and communication as Autism Spectrum Disorders (ASD).

In the U.S., 1 in 150 children are autistic, according to the Centers for Disease Control. That adds up to almost 1.5 million people in the United States. In the Canary Islands there is 1 autistic child per 166 live births. The number of people diagnosed with autism has increased dramatically since the 1980's. ASDs are more common than were once believed and are considered conditions of urgent public health concern.

Arquímides Fernández-Valdés, from School of Psychology at La Laguna University in the Canary Islands, Spain, states that: "The difficulty in managing autism resides in the lack of knowledge about its cause. The great majority of specialists understand that there are no environmental, educational or social factors that are thought to contribute to the development of autism. If we only knew the reason, we might make great advances."

Brain Research in Autism

The various modern techniques that either directly or indirectly image the structure, function and pharmacology of the brain allow the monitoring of the state of the brain in different moments. They show hypoperfusion in the brain of the autistic patients. This poor blood delivery is mostly noted in areas responsible for communication and social interaction, and this could be the reason for typical focusing in the "self". Notably, the functional magnetic resonance imaging of a normal brain shows a compensatory rise in cerebral blood flow when the person is performing some tasks. When autistic persons are doing the same task, they often lack this increase.

The cause of this hypoperfusion in autistic children is still unknown, but it might be linked with inflammation in the brain. One study published in 2005 showed this phenomenon in autistic patients. Another study demonstrated evidence of cerebral edema (swelling) in autistic children. This means that there is the accumulation of liquids in the space between cells, so that oxygen needs to cross a longer distance from the capillaries to neurons in autistic children. When cells lack oxygen, this state is called hypoxia. Hypoperfusion, inflammation, edema and hypoxia all create poor conditions for metabolism in the autistic brain, which, to some extent, can explain the behavioral difficulties in these children.

Other possible mechanisms of autism can involve a mitochondrial dysfunction. Mitochondria are tiny power stations in each cell. They produce the energy that keeps us alive. Several published papers pertaining to autistic patients, called "case reports" (a detailed report of the symptoms, signs, diagnosis, treatment, and follow-up of an individual patient), and "case series" (several patients) have shown abnormal levels of certain metabolites that prove mitochondrial dysfunction in autistic patients. Because of the fact that energy production is the main function of mitochondria, a dysfunction in mitochondria always diminishes energy metabolism.

HBO for Autism

HBO is the best method to overcome the effects of cerebral hypoperfusion, thus eliminating hypoxia. HBO provides more oxygen to the brain and at the same time it is a powerful tool to reduce cerebral edema. Inflammation also comes under control with hyperbaric oxygen. Dr. Daniel A. Rossignol, at the International Child Development

Resource Center in Melbourne, Florida, U.S., showed a decline in C-reactive protein, which is known as an inflammation marker, in autistic patients. In a group of children treated with HBO this drop was of almost 90%. Finally, the effect of HBO discovered by Dr. Steve Thom at the University of Philadelphia in mobilizing stem cells in the bone marrow and increasing its quantity in circulation, might also take part in reversing some brain disorders in these children.

HBO improves the mitochondrial function; furthermore, it protects mitochondria from deterioration, when compared with normal oxygen level and pressure. For this reason, Dr. Rossignol thinks that HBO might improve the relative mitochondrial dysfunction found in autistic children.

How Are Autistic Children Treated?

In others chapters we have mentioned the pressure at which patients with different pathologies are treated: at 2.0 ATA for wound healing or almost 3.0 ATA for patients with carbon monoxide poisoning. The injured brain needs very low pressures. Dr. Neubauer proposed and used 1.5 ATA, but in the last years only 28-30% of oxygen at 1.3 ATA seemed to improve some chronic neurological conditions.

Outcome of HBO Application in Autistic Children

Dr. Rossignol noted that younger children have more significant improvement in clinical outcome than older children. This observation is matched by reports from Dr. Neubauer and Dr. Golden published in 2002 in the International Journal of Neuroscience. Probably, HBO can improve future cerebral development in younger children overcoming the effect of brain hypoperfusion. Clinical improvement was observed in diverse areas including irritability, social withdrawal, hyperactivity, motivation, speech and cognitive functions.

In 2009, a randomized controlled multi-centered study of 62 children by Dr. Rossignol was published by BMC Pediatrics that demonstrated that HBO at 1.3 ATA is safe and efficacious in children with autism compared to a control group.

But Dr. Jepson and coworkers at the Thoughtful House Center for Children, in Austin, Texas, using this protocol in 16 children with autistic profile did not find any improvement in them after 40 HBO sessions.

So, outcomes vary between the different studies.

The Undersea and Hyperbaric Medical Society, known as UHMS, lists approvals for reimbursement of HBOT for certain diagnoses in hospitals and clinics. The use of HBOT in autism is still not approved for reimbursement by the UHMS Hyperbaric Oxygen Therapy Committee. But there is a special UHMS position paper in relation to HBO treatment of autistic spectrum disorders, which states that at this time (2010), the UHMS cannot recommend the routine treatment of ASD with HBO outside appropriate comparative research protocols. The UHMS is proposing to assist in the development and conduction of suitable studies with high methodological rigor in this area.

To Treat or Not to Treat Autistic Children with HBO

Autistic children present restrictive and repetitive behavior. This condition was traditionally considered as "static", without probability of improvement, in spite of many different treatment approaches: educational, psychological, clinical, musical therapy, equine therapy, etc.

The parents of autistic children face many difficulties. The first one is the impact of the disease, but a second and very important one is "What should I do with my child?"

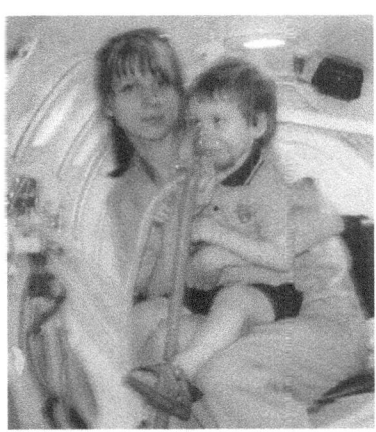

It is difficult to convince a child not to remove the mask.

Many parents are seeking alternative therapies; the foremost being HBOT. Why? Up to now there is only one controlled randomized trial in addition to others studies with less scientific rigor that also show favorable outcomes of this method in ASD. Besides, there are other papers that report an improvement in cerebral functions in healthy children treated in hyperbaric chamber. They showed a higher level of attention, reaction time, and word search.

When I am asked by parents if it is worthwhile to treat their autistic child with hyperbaric oxygen, I consent only under the condition that the attending neurologist agree with this therapy and will evaluate the outcome as a third party. Obviously, the patient will be checked for any contraindications.

As a rule, the parents see more improvements in their children than the physicians. Accuracy in protocol selection, close observation of each patient and working as a team with the neurologist are the keys for success of this treatment.

We have treated a few autistic children. We asked the family to write down the changes in their behavior and look for a third party evaluation from a school teacher or psychologist.

The psychologist of Thomas reported that after 37 HBO sessions in addition to rehabilitation treatment, his behavior improved progressively, although it still varies. Thomas is able to hold his attention for longer periods, maintains better relations with adults, doesn't take off his clothes any more, has learned to put on his shoes and tie the laces and appears friendlier, as observed also by our staff.

Conclusion

With the favorable results observed with HBO application and facing the lack of others methods with good outcomes in children with ASD, parents might decide on the use of hyperbaric chamber as a means to improve some aspects of autistic behavior in their children.

Cerebral Palsy

Cerebral palsy is a collective term used to refer to any one of a number of neurological disorders that appear in infancy or early childhood and permanently affect body movement and posture. Besides motor impairment, the sensory sphere could be damaged; some patients present at the same time epilepsy, learning difficulties, and behavioral problems. There are an estimated 2 children with cerebral palsy per 1000 live births.

Clinical Presentation

Cerebral palsy is a condition characterized by a variety of symptoms; its clinical picture is very diverse. While one child with severe cerebral palsy might be unable to walk and need lifelong care, another might be only slightly awkward and require no special assistance because of a mild level of cerebral palsy.

The majority of children with cerebral palsy are born with it, although it may not be detected until months or years later. The first signs of cerebral palsy usually appear before a child reaches 3 years of age although more common from 12 to 18 months from birth, when it becomes clear that the child fails to develop such basic motor functions as sitting upright, maintaining the sitting position, crawling and kneeling, and standing and walking.

Children also can show alterations in motor functions, such as asymmetry in movements or unusual muscle stiffness or floppiness. This stiffness is called spasticity and it is common in 75% of patients. Children with concomitant epilepsy have seizures of different severity.

Developmental Implications

Cerebral palsy provokes different developmental disabilities. Altered motor function disturbs the child's capacity to explore actively the world around him or her and to learn it. The lack of independence creates social consequences of this disease.

Cerebral palsy cannot be cured, but the aim of therapy is the improvement of functional abilities that facilitate independence and quality of life. One of the goals in cerebral palsy treatment is the reduction of spasticity or stiffness in different muscle groups. This stiffness can be very painful, distort posture and may require surgery.

Treatment

Treatment includes physical and occupational therapy, speech therapy, drugs to control seizures, to relax muscle spasms, and to alleviate pain; surgery to correct anatomical abnormalities or release tight muscles; braces, wheelchairs and rolling walkers; and communication aids such as computers with attached voice synthesizers.

New trends in treatment include low intensity electrical stimulation of the muscles that does not produce movement in response but acts as a stimulus. Another method is the use of a therapy suit to promote independent mobility. In both cases the effectiveness of the treatments is not supported by solid clinical trial.

HBO also is used in cerebral palsy treatment.

How Can Hyperbaric Oxygen Help in Cerebral Palsy?

Not all cerebral palsy patients are necessarily candidates for HBO. The benefit from hyperbaric oxygen is expected in cases associated with a traumatic brain injury or with a toxic, hypoxic or anoxic encephalopathy. These conditions are known under the collective term BITHAE (from the first letters of these words). The damaged brain areas enter in a specific functional state called "ischemic penumbra" and the damaged neurons turn to "idling". The concept of ischemic penumbra was explained in a previous chapter.

The "idling" neurons are viable, but electrically non-functional. This is potentially recoverable tissue. How can physicians prove that the state of these neurons can be reversed?

Dr. Neubauer was the first to use SPECT (single photon emission computerized tomography), which allows the visualization of active cells because they take in and store a tracer used in this method. After HBO the "idling" neurons become active and begin to store the tracer. The change in SPECT results is parallel to the clinical improvement. Dr. Neubauer demonstrated benefits from HBO in the motor skills of his patients, attention, alertness, concentration, vision and verbal and non-verbal communications.

Over the course of 30 years Dr. Neubauer treated many patients but he did not conduct any controlled randomized study. Understanding the necessity of such a study, he explained its difficulties. First, there is an ethical issue in not providing treatment to half the patients. Second, the variability in clinical pictures, brain areas injured, severity of defects and highly individualized nature of this disease make it very difficult to select groups for a randomized double blind study.

In 1999, Dr. Montgomery and colleagues from McGill University in Montreal, Canada, reported improvement in motor skills of patients and also a reduction of spasticity. They observed improvement in sitting, crawling and kneeling, standing and walking, running and jumping in 25 children from 3 to 8 years of age with cerebral palsy after receiving 20 HBO treatments at 1.75 ATA for 60 minutes.

These preliminary results justified a larger prospective controlled study. Such a study was conducted by practically the same team of Canadian researchers guided by Dr. Collet and published in 2001 in one of the most prestigious journals – "Lancet". They divided 111 children from 3 to 11 years of age in two groups: one received hyperbaric oxygen at 1.75 ATA and another room air at 1.3 ATA, which corresponds to breathing 28% of oxygen at normal atmospheric pressure, in total 40 treatments. Both groups improved their motor functions, self-control and auditory attention, speech and memory as well.

There are some important issues in this study. First, the control group also received more oxygen than the normal content of oxygen in the air. Nowadays, with the development of "low" and "extra-low" protocol, 28% of oxygen seems to work in the control group. Second, one of the main side effects was ear barotrauma, which was suffered by almost half of the children in the hyperbaric oxygen group (27 of 57) and only a quarter (15 of 57) in the control group. This complication could have affected the outcome of the study. In the previous study by Montgomery, pressure equalization tubes were inserted in the ears of 13 children to avoid ear barotrauma.

> **Aylen with her prizes**
>
>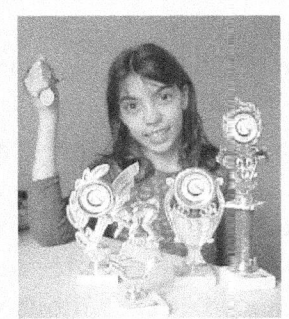
>
> We have treated a 9-year-old girl with cerebral palsy that appeared after the child suffered encephalomyelitis at age 3. Her tongue was paralyzed, and she suffered from shortness of breath because of difficulties in swallowing saliva.
>
> Although she received HBO after 6 years of physical and rehabilitation therapy that reached a plateau in her performance, her improvement was very pronounced — she overcame the swallowing problems —, thus bettering the rhythm of respiration and even won prizes in swimming

HBO in cerebral palsy treatment is used in other countries. Since 2001, Dr. Arun Mukherjee in India has been conducting a controlled study of HBO therapy in brain injured children. It includes cerebral palsy and autism. The protocol for HBO therapy comprises 40 sessions at 1.75 ATA and 1.5 ATA with 100% oxygen during 90 minutes each. The control group receives hyperbaric air at 1.25 ATA. He observed cognitive improvement in treated children. This improvement is permanent, while spasticity improves only when the protocol of standard therapy is repeated regularly. This study is still ongoing.

Another group of Indian physicians – Dr. Sheila S. Mathai and colleagues in Mumbai -reported improvement in gross motor function measures and in speech in children with cerebral palsy after 90 HBO sessions.

Dr. José Machado in San Paulo, Brazil, found that in 218 out of 230 (94.78%) patients with spastic form of cerebral palsy, there was a clear reduction of spasticity. The follow-up of patients over a period of 6 or more months after HBOT showed the persistent reduction of spasticity and better motor control. In addition, parents reported other improvements, such as enhanced balance, the child becoming more attentive and more "intelligent," and a reduced frequency of convulsions and episodes of bronchitis.

One of the noticeable effects of hyperbaric oxygen therapy in neurological patients is the reduction of spasticity. Is it enough to justify HBO application? The outstanding neurologist William Landau who was listed in the Best Doctors in America wrote: "There need be no apology for tackling only a symptom rather than an etiology; the misery of these patients cannot wait."

Conclusion

There are no controlled clinical studies that prove the use of HBO in cases of cerebral palsy, but there is some benefit that could be explained by the activation of "idling" neurons. The proof of the beneficial effects of hyperbaric oxygen in the injured brain is in the SPECT images, which show improvement in cerebral perfusion. The idea of Dr. Neubauer was to include SPECT imaging as a routine procedure in the treatment of these patients. That documentation could add the scientific rigor to the clinical research and finally help finding the best oxygen dosage and protocol for treatment.

The use of HBO in cerebral palsy is still not approved for reimbursement by the UHMS Hyperbaric Oxygen Therapy Committee.

Nowadays the decision of HBO treatment of patients with cerebral palsy is in the hands of parents and neurologists. It seems that the best protocol for cerebral palsy treatment with the inclusion of HBO has yet to be found; meanwhile the accumulation of scientifically analyzed results allows us to seek a better care for this group of children.

> "There need be no apology for tackling only a symptom rather than an etiology; the misery of these patients cannot wait."
> *Doctor William Landau.*

Contraindications, Side effects and Complications

Contraindications to hiperbaric oxygen therapy are associated with three factors: changes of external pressure to which the patient's body is subjected, high oxygen concentration that the patient inhales and the reduced and closed space inside the chamber.

Changes to external pressure

Patients with certain pulmonary diseases and conditions: asymptomatic air cysts or blebs in the lungs, which look like air filled sacks in X-ray, may have problems during compression and decompression. These sacks may rupture producing pneumothorax, or collection of air in the pleural cavity, which can be life threatening. That is why we ask for a chest X-ray before HBO treatment. Also caverns (typical in patients with tuberculosis), abscesses, and pneumonia can be dangerous in the sense of conserving integrity of the lung tissue in the face of variations of chamber pressure. But if the patient already has pneumothorax and needs HBO as a life-saving measure, she or he can be treated after the surgical relief of pneumothorax. This situation sometimes occurs in divers. Upper respiratory infections predispose to nose and throat congestion, that cause difficulties in controlling middle ear pressure that in turn trigger barotrauma of the ears or paranasal sinus cavities.

If the pressure of air trapped in the middle ear is not equal to external pressure, the patient first feels discomfort, then pain because of tympanic membrane displacement, which, if not resolved, may be enough to its rupture (barotrauma). When the pressure inside the middle ear or paranasal sinuses is lower than the external pressure, a relative vacuum occurs, attracting lymph and blood, thus causing inflammation. The same processes happen when landing an airplane or diving.

This effect occurs only during compression and decompression. We teach our patients that simple swallowing or using other maneuvers, when the chamber changes pressure, can equalize the internal and external ear pressures. However, if a patient has sinus polyps, development's anomalies, a cold's congestion, or his external ear canal is occluded with earwax, barotrauma may also happen with pain and hemorrhages. That's why we ask these patients to consult an otolaryngologist before HBO treatment.

High Oxygen Concentration

We can breathe 100% pure oxygen at normal atmospheric pressure for several days without problems. At a pressure of 2 atmospheres we can inhale pure oxygen during no more than 24 hours. At 3 atmospheres this period is cut down to some hours and at 5 atmospheres to a few minutes. All the protocols in hyperbaric oxygen therapy are established beneath these limits. If these rules are violated, seizures might be present, to which patients with epilepsy and major individual sensitivity to oxygen are more prone.

Reduced and Closed Space

Claustrophobic people are not the best candidates to enter the chamber.

-oOo-

All these contraindications are relative. If the treatment can save the patient's life, for example, as in a case of gas gangrene or carbon monoxide poisoning, the conditions that limit the use of the hyperbaric chamber can be adjusted. An epileptic patient should receive anticonvulsant drugs before treatment is initiated, the pneumothorax should be drained and in an unconscious person that is not able to equalize pressure in the middle ear, a tiny incision may be created in the eardrum, a special medical procedure called miryngotomy.

Only patients with precise diagnosis should be subject to the hyperbaric oxygen treatment. For example, a patient with uncontrolled high fever of unknown origin should not receive HBO treatments. If the cause of the fever is determined and the necessity of HBO application is justified, the fever should be reduced below 100.5 °F before placing the patient in the chamber, because it may predispose to oxygen seizures.

These are not Contraindications:

Tumors. Although tumors do not constitute contraindications, HBO should be postponed if the patient receives chemotherapeutic agents, such as doxorubicin or cisplatin, and reconsidered if the patient has received bleomycin.

Pregnancy. For decades pregnancy was considered an absolute contraindication to HBO treatment. As in diving, it was thought that bubble formation could damage the fetus, and also that hyperbaric oxygen might stimulate premature circulation changes in the fetus. Extensive research in the Soviet Union, in which women in all stages of pregnancy when treated with HBO giving birth to normal children that stayed in good health, put an end to these

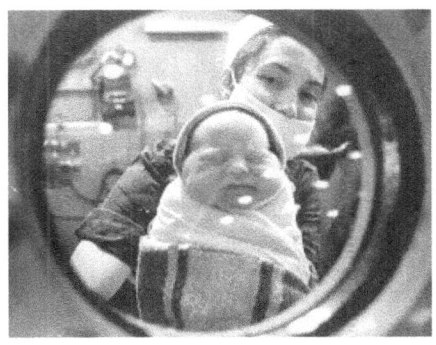

First baby born inside a hyperbaric chamber at the Moscow Barocenter. His mother suffered acute myocardial infarction at 36 weeks of pregnancy- Both were saved. Courtesy: Professor S.N. Efuny M.D., Ph.D.

fears. The lack of negative effects of HBO on fetus and neonates has been later reported by some Western authors.

Implantable Pacemakers. These modern devices resist environmental pressure changes.

Side Effects

Some patients, after receiving 30 or more treatments in hyperbaric chamber develop transitory myopia. They report that their presbyopia improves. Generally, lens refractive changes disappear in a short time. In some patients with multiple sclerosis treated with hundreds of HBO treatments the appearance of cataracts in previously transparent lens has been observed. But it doesn't appear when the total of HBO treatments is kept below 150. It has also been suggested that preexisting cataracts mature more rapidly with HBO, although this has not been proved.

Complications

Hypoglycemia. Hypoglycemia can precipitate transpiration, weakness, disorientation and loss of conscious-

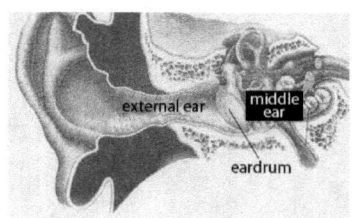

Inside the hyperbaric chamber a patient needs to equalize the pressure in the middle ear with the external air pressure.

ness. Diabetic patients should monitor blood glucose and receive proper nutrients one or one and a half hours before treatment in order to maintain normal levels of sugar in the blood. People who use insulin are at a higher risk of hypoglycemia. Both insulin and oral hypoglycemic drugs (agents, medication) become more effective with repetitive HBO treatments.

Seizures. Convulsions may occur as a result of hypoglycemia. A patient can also have them on account of his or her neurologic disorders. Patients with a history of seizures should consult a neurologist and undergo hyperbaric oxygen treatment only if they continue taking their routine anticonvulsant medications in an updated dose.

Conclusion

In actual practice, there are no absolute contraindications to hyperbaric oxygen therapy. Side effects and complications are very unusual. However, patients receiving HBO therapy need keen attention at every moment because their general state of health could be very fragile. The hyperbaric physician can advise against taking this treatment if the probability of improvement is poor. The decision to continue or to suspend the treatment depends on the clinical outcome in each patient. Any decision should be consulted with the physician that initially indicated this therapy.

Anti-Aging

Most hyperbaric medicine specialists refuse to speak in public about the efficacy of this branch of medical practice in slowing down the aging process. They believe that doing so may cast doubt on the benefits of this therapy to cure numerous diseases and conditions.

But facts are stubborn things. These same hyperbaric physicians (I am personally acquainted with some of them) subject themselves to hyperbaric oxygen (HBO) treatment. And many of them are not longer in their most flourishing period of Lfe. They report that this treatment enhances both their physical and mental performance.

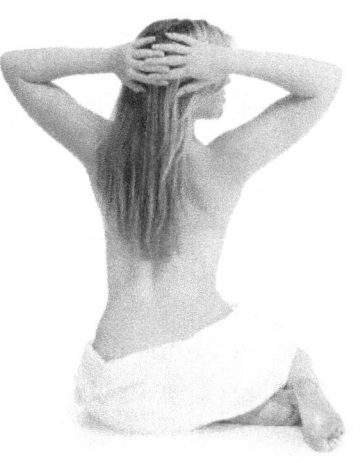

Some physicians think that hyperbaric oxygen can revitalize their elderly patients in body and mind. As skin gets toned up, its elasticity is greatly improved and wrinkles vanish.

It is worth mentioning that in the 19th century in large cities of Europe such as London, Brussels, Vienna, Amsterdam, Berlin and Milan, it was popular to do "air bathing" at specially designed "Pneumatic Centers" (1837-1877). There the people stayed for a while in hermetic chambers with compressed air. Many of them became addicted because they felt better and with more energy when taking these "baths."

With the development of hyperbaric medicine physicians have found that patients treated with HBO for specific diseases also improve their general health and well-being: they sleep more soundly and do not get as tired as before. And nails and skin look more vital and bright.

Is it worth treating healthy people who want to improve their well-being, appearance, vitality and quality of life? In my opinion, yes. Aging, both natural and induced by stress or by the sun, is associated with a decrease in oxygen levels. Oxygen has become the latest trend in beauty products, for example, oxygen creams. It is assumed that skin moisturizes and rejuvenates with the use of these modern cosmetics.

With age what happens to cells? The function of each cell is codified, each one is programmed with what it has to do. For example, pancreatic beta cells produce insulin. Aging and diseases are both associated with programming errors.

Continuing with the example, insulin becomes modified when it is interpreted in error, as if a spelling mistake was made, and the final product is "insuline". Some errors are small and so the sense of the word or phrase is not lost. Other errors produce a substance that cannot perform its function. This process of making mistakes is permanent and our body has mechanisms to fix them.

Why do these errors happen? Apparently we can blame environmental pollution: chemically aggressive substances and the ultraviolet radiation, which induce the formation of so-called "free radicals". A free radical is a very active atom or group of atoms that contains an unpaired electron, which has a great capacity to bind. The unpaired electrons cause radicals to be chemically highly reactive. It's like a blind man running around in a crowd with a knife. And so these radicals roam our body trying to steal an electron from stable molecules to achieve electrochemical stability.

When the free radical has succeeded in stealing the needed electron the stable molecule that has given up the electron is converted in turn into a free radical lacking one electron, initiating a chain reaction that can destroy many cells.

The free radicals are not essentially "bad". As a matter of fact, our own body generates free radicals in adequate quantities to fight against bacteria and viruses. Free radicals play an important role in human physiology. For example, superoxide and nitric oxide regulate many biological processes, such as controlling vascular tone. Such radicals can even be messengers in a phenomenon dubbed redox signaling. They also contribute to the renewal of body structures: degrading old formations and synthesizing new molecules. Once they have done their job, our own antioxidant system neutralizes them easily. For this purpose our organism produces several special substances. These substances can lend free radicals the electron they lack without themselves losing their chemical stability. The process of losing an electron is called "oxidation"

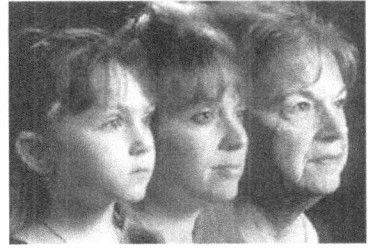

in chemical language, thus these substances are called "antioxidants".

A calculation of the harmful action of free radicals yielded a result as 104 daily modifications in each cell. While everything is fine in the organism, these processes do not lead to disease because the body has a high capacity for repair, a kind of maintenance in which these same antioxidants are taking part. But if they stop working properly, there is a possibility that a tiny part of these modifications escape repair. This is the beginning of a biological process of uncontrolled growth (cancer) or degeneration – the essence of aging. How could this damage be prevented? By enhancing the antioxidant power of the organism. The consumption of antioxidants such as beta-carotene (vitamin A precursor), tocopherol (vitamin E) and ascorbic acid (vitamin C) was proposed as a solution to the problem. These antioxidants are powerful; and are present in foods or taken in tablets.

From the 1980's large scale use of these protective substances, or antioxidants, as micronutrients to prevent or slow down the development of cardiovascular disease and cancer began, with great expectations. However, the results of epidemiologic and population studies have been disappointing and not demonstrating a beneficial effect. Limited data suggest there may be adverse consequences of antioxidant supplementation, especially in patients with cancer.

Why did this happen? We go back to the free radicals. They are part of our normal biochemistry. Up to 5% of all oxygen that enters a cell change into free radicals, or reactive oxygen species (ROS). These are produced not as by-products but as regular components that participate in cell metabolism "with full rights". Reactive oxygen species turned out to be even more important than first thought. They are indispensable as they transmit signals. They propagate messages from one cell to another "telling" them what to do, and telling the nucleus of cell which substances it should produce. They are protagonists in the main processes of regulation.

> Patients who are treated in the hyperbaric chamber because of some approved indication find an improvement of their general state of health, and overall appearance, as well as their psychic, physical, and sexual performance.

Many substances in our organism are known to need specific receptors in the cell membrane in order to work, for example, catecholamines, insulin, and other hormones, neurotransmitters, etc. But the majority of external agents: lack of oxygen, high or low temperatures, etc. do not have specific receptors. How does the cell recognize these factors? By means of reactive oxygen species.

Inside the cell there is a protein sensitive to oxidation upon which ROS act. The signal is then transmitted through well-known routes, which are common to both specific and non-specific receptors, reaching the nucleus. The nucleus uses this information to begin producing protective substances, adequate for each case.

There are 3 options for the oxidative signal: it could be weak, moderate or strong.

1. With a weak oxidative signal available antioxidants are spent so that new ones not need to be synthesized. The general state of the cell doesn't change.

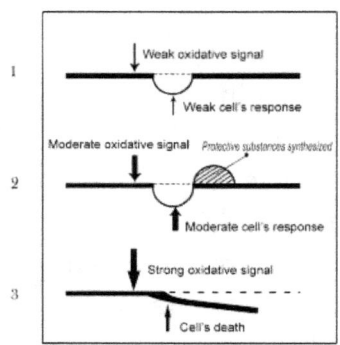

Options for the oxidative signal:
1 - weak, 2 – moderate, 3 - strong.

2. With a moderate oxidative signal an important response is generated: a synthesis of protective substances. And for a few days the cell has a slight excess of antioxidant defenses. This ensures protection against not only oxidants but also other agents that in turn can be much more powerful. It's a response to" training".

Now we suppose that this is the manner of how is activated the response against hypoxia, stress, injuries from ischemia-reperfusion and other situations in which the organism may or may not survive.

3. But when an extraordinarily strong oxidative signal presents, or free radicals enter the cell in great amount, the antioxidant systems of the cell probably cannot handle it and the protection against oxidation might be overcome. At this time exogenous antioxidants are needed or the cell may perish.

Hence, one of the universal defense mechanisms of the cell is the synthesis of antioxidants. In training with free radicals of moderate strength the cell becomes saturated with protective molecules against different harmful agents. The more protective substances, the greater the probability of survival.

Now it is clear that endogenous antioxidants, those produced by the cell itself, are more important, than antioxidants consumed as additives in our food. Antioxidants taken as pills let the cell in relax, they block the tran-

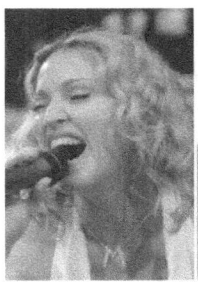 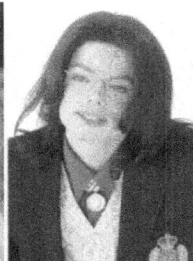 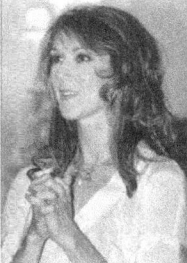 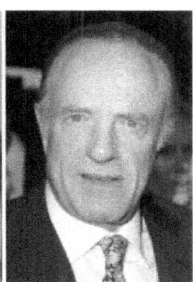

scription of factors that activate the genetic apparatus of the cell. At this point it is clear why efforts to treat cardiovascular diseases and cancer with exogenous antioxidants failed. Thousands of pills taken did not lead to a decrease in mortality or morbidity.

Another option offers the hyperbaric chamber: it stimulates the generation of endogenous antioxidants, some specific substances, mostly enzymes. This phenomenon is observed in patients under HBO treatment. Unlike antioxidants consumed by mouth, these appear directly in the place where they are needed, and in the amounts required, and they do not block the routes of transmission of signals.

Madonna and Celine Dion are known around the world. They have a youthful look and seem to be immune to the wearing down occasioned by time. Madonna revealed to a German magazine the secret of her eternal youthful appearance: she habitually uses a hyperbaric chamber to look and feel her best.

We still recall Michael Jackson, whose photo in 1986 in the magazine "National Enquirer" became famous. In this photo Michael Jackson is seen sleeping in a hyperbaric chamber to delay aging. His untimely death does not take away merits from the hyperbaric chamber, it actually highlights them. Who knows what would have become of him if he had not stopped being a fanatic of sleeping in the chamber rather than taking pills.

Celine Dion and actor James Caan are convinced that sessions in the hyperbaric oxygen chamber improve sleep, concentration, and vitality. Tiger Woods has said he has received oxygen treatment in a hyperbaric chamber. It has been reported that Fidel Castro receives hyperbaric treatment periodically at the CIMEQ Hospital in Havana.

One effect of vital importance achieved in the field of hyperbaric oxygen therapy is the "magic" of helping us stay mentally alert, to appear and feel younger and more agile, and to delay aging and senility.

Occasionally we receive "patients" which should in fact be called "clients", as they do not present an established pathology. Generally, they are high executives that work in stress environments and desire to improve their performance, mood and stamina. And they achieve these results in the hyperbaric chamber.

There are millions of people with mental and physical disabilities due to age. The proportion of seniors grows each year all over the world. Any treatment that can prolong their ability to participate in a normal life, what is now called "quality of life", is very important.

How long do results last? Much longer than hairstyling or beauty treatment. Generally, between six and nine months, after which it is necessary to submit to the therapy again.

Jules Verne gave a quick end to the Doctor Ox's Experiment. If he had prolonged the story, we would have found out how the old people rejuvenated in Quiquendone.

REIMERS SYSTEMS, INC.
www.ReimersSystems.com

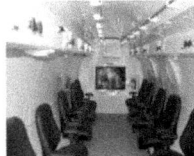
Multiplace Systems

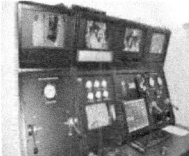
Touch Screen Console

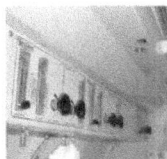
Hood Drivers

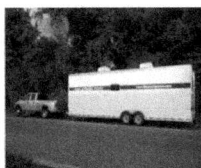
Mobile Facilities

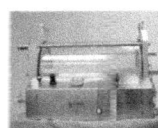
Research Chambers

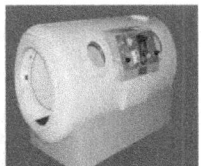
RSI 4200 Monoplace

PRODUCTS:
- Multiplace clinical HBO chambers of any size including segmented and self contained systems
- Altitude physiology training chambers
- Research chambers
- Mobile hyperbaric units
- Veterinary chambers
- Breathing simulators for performance testing
- Manifolds and gas selection panels
- Gas selection panels and manifolds
- TCOM and utility penetrators
- TV/DVD setups for monoplace and multiplace
- Air ventilation conversion for monoplace chambers
- Hood drivers
- And more......

SERVICES:
- Oxygen service solutions to fit any site
- Site design and development
- Turnkey site installation services
- Field re-window services
- Overhaul, relocation and maintenance
- Operations procedures, safety surveys
- CAD design and conversion
- Fabrication design and drawing review
- Appraisals

QUALITY PRE-OWNED EQUIPMENT:
Visit our HCI affiliate at:
www.Hyperbaric-Clearinghouse.com

Reimers Systems, Inc.
www.ReimersSystems.com
info@ReimersSystems.com

8210-D Cinder Bed Road
Lorton, VA 22079
Phone: 703-952-0240
Fax: 703-952-0244

www.ingramcontent.com/pod-product-compliance
Lightning Source LLC
Chambersburg PA
CBHW051717170526
45167CB00002B/689